Nursing Chose Me

Called to an Art of Compassion

Dr. Karen Reichel Smith
Doctorate of Nursing Practice

ISBN-10:151737341X
ISBN-13:978-1517375416
Printed by CreateSpace, Charleston S.C.
Available from Amazon.com

All of the stories are based on real people and situations.
All names have been changed.

DEDICATION

To Chuck
When there is no talking, the walking is there.
Together we're content to be.

CONTENTS

ACKNOWLEDGMENTS

There is a sea of nameless faces, patients who for a brief moment in time put their trust in me to keep them safe from harm and free from pain. They allowed me to "practice" nursing on them. They have given my life meaning and purpose.

I want to thank the millions of nurses who put their heart and soul into the care of patients every hour of every day, year after year, crisis after crisis, shortage after shortage, with or without breaks, brow beaten defenders of patient needs… my soul mates.

And with all my love, I would like to thank my spouse, my friends and family for their editing guidance and ongoing encouragement.

PROLOGUE

Shortly after I began my nursing career, I sat down with the intention to write a novel about what it was like to be a bedside nurse. I spent the summer writing, polishing and rewriting it while the details were still fresh in my mind. I declared the book "finished" to my family at the conclusion of that season.

Every couple of years and every career shift necessitated the addition of another chapter and another summer of writing, polishing and rewriting after which I would declare the book "really finished" to my family.

This book, like me, may have started out to be just a story of a bedside nurse, but that turned out to be only the beginning of my journey in nursing amidst a whirlwind of technological changes in an ever changing health care system.

As I reflect back over several decades of experiences in many different settings, one theme emerges. Suffering and pain are the immutable part of the human experience. Therefore the need for compassionate care transcends time. From the days of Florence Nightingale to an age where "care" robots float down the hall, there will always be a wrinkly faced patient lying alone and scared waiting for the nurse.

A loving touch, a listening ear, a gentle word - will never go out of date.

I believe that behind the computer screens, next to the flashing and beeping monitors, draped in miles of IV tubing and weighed down with bags of medications, there are nurses, who like me, chose nursing to make a difference.

This is my true story, "finished…for now."

"Many are the plans in a man's heart,
but a man's steps are directed by the Lord."
Proverbs 19:21

PART ONE:

NURSING IN THE TRENCHES

1

Any 21 year old could do this with 3O years experience...

Memories of that first day on the job are quite vivid. Frightened would be an understatement. I watched as the other nurses hung their coats and chatted with each other, noticeably at ease with their established roles. To them it was just another day. To me, it was evidence that I had finally made it and I wanted nothing better than to run home and pretend that I hadn't graduated yet from nursing school.

I became a nurse by accident. My parents thought, because I was a girl, that nursing was a better career choice than the doctor I had dreamed of becoming from the age of five. "It's like being a doctor, but you don't have to be in school as long. This way you can have a family."

I went along my parents' guidance, mistakenly believing that at the baccalaureate level, nursing was just a "major", like biology or chemistry, and that I could "use" this towards medical school when I was done. I discovered during my senior year of college that none of my nursing courses counted "academically" towards the medical school requirements. So, faced with the prospect of having to spend another year in college taking plant biology and a different chemistry course, I reluctantly donned the nursing cap and white uniform, took the exam, and found myself standing in the line of RNs, two courses and a lifetime away from my childhood dream. I was totally oblivious to the career path I had surreptitiously embarked upon!

When I first graduated eons ago, licensed nurses provided most of the patient care, while "technicians" worked in the engineering department of the hospital. Holistic care was practiced, not preached. I accepted a RN position on 5 North, a medical-surgical unit in a community hospital. I was assigned to the day shift, with rotation to evening and nights as needed. They needed it often.

Walking down the lusterless sea green painted hallway there was no mistaking you were in a hospital. Like most hospitals back then, there was only an occasional motel grade picture breaking the monotony of the dimly lit corridors. Each room produced its own mix of smells from a brew of urine, feces, sick breath, cafeteria food and ammonia based hospital sanitizers, emanating into the hallway as you passed.

The nurses' station was halfway down the hall with a secretary's desk in front, shielded from visitors by a three foot high piece of Plexiglas on the front and side that looked like a bookie stall. Several phones, charts and notebooks scattered on top of the long desk in the station left little free space for the bustling nurses. There was one small desk area labeled "Reserved for the Doctors" with a bookcase over top housing a tattered collection of donated textbooks for the nurses. The bathroom, labeled "Nurses Only", inferred "ladies" only. The medication room looked like a one-person kitchen without the stove. The drawers, refrigerator and cabinets were filled with stock medicines, syringes and needles.

Across the hall were two large utility rooms. The "clean" one contained a large supplies cart and cabinets stuffed to capacity with boxes and bags of new or recycled medical equipment. The "dirty" one housed the garbage cans, the bedpan hopper, where filled bedpans were dumped and steam cleaned, cleaning supplies, dirty equipment and samples waiting for lab pick-up. Both rooms were totally devoid of decoration.

On this first day, a friendly face found me and invited me to stand closer so that I could hear the morning report. My preceptor, Carol, who was my assigned buddy for orientation purposes, was busy taking charge of the unit for the day. I stood in awe at her level of comfort with such tremendous responsibility. She prepared herself at the helm.

"Are these pre-ops ready? Consents signed? Labs on the chart?" as she quickly flipped the pages of the patient chart. "Where's the sterilization consent?" She turned to the girl at her side, "Donna, you better get that done now, they could call any minute. I don't need Dr. Rasper breathing down my neck today."

Turning back to the night nurse, "How much is in that IV?"

The night nurse scrambled through her notes, "400cc at O-600. It's an 18, but it's positional. I marked it on the cover of the chart."

"Thanks. How about allergies?"

"None."

"Okay, let's get on with report. It looks like it's gonna be a busy one!" Carol spun around to look at the staff who had gathered behind her. She spotted me. We had met once before. "Hi Karen! Welcome to Five North. Looks like I'm not going to be able to work next to you today like we planned. The head nurse called in sick so I've got to take charge today. I'll be around if you get stuck. Did you see your assignment?"

Numb with fright, I shook my head no.

"You've got these five patients here. Only two are completes, so you should be okay."

I choked, the most patients I had ever had in school was two at a time.

Carol added, "Leah can help you out if you can't find something."

Leah, an elderly, overweight LPN with a cigarette hanging from her mouth heard her name.

"I'm not doing anything else today. My back's sore."

"Leah, this is Karen, she is a new grad. I just offered your help if she can't find something."

Leah snuffed out her cigarette and rolled her eyes. "Yeah, right," she huffed, then left the nurses' station.

Carol chuckled, seeing my face. "She's really not so bad. Don't let her scare you! "

The night nurse began a whirlwind of commentary that left me totally perplexed. My tension mounted as they neared my patients.

"Mr. Sabatini, patient of DMSV in Room 14. In for a revision of a cabbage. History of 2 anterior wall MI's. Status Post Turp 2 years ago, PVD, and ASHD."

My mind rummaged through the content stored from each Baccalaureate course I had taken in attempt to decode the report in progress to no avail.

"He has an IV in his left antecubital. Pre-op for tomorrow. VSS. IV of D5 Half Normal at KVO. 600 up."

"Any chest pain?" Carol asked.

"None on nights. Evenings gave him two nitros at 1800."

I scratched down "pre-op, IV, and chest pain" on my paper. The rest had been gibberish. I would have to look at the Kardex information myself later.

"Next is Mrs. Smythe in 15A. She is one of MOP's. Had a T-A-H-B-S-O three days ago. Foley out at 6. Hasn't voided yet. Vitals were 130 over 70, 84, 12, and 99.5 at 12, 120 over 60, 82, 16, 98.8 at 6. Passing flatus. Dressings D and I."

I wrote down "15A Smythe, check voiding, foley out at 6, 99.5? gas, dressing?" This woman could speak at the speed of light. I had more gaps than information from this report. My armpits became noticeably wet and I felt as though I would get sick. If only I knew what diseases my patients had, I would have a starting point. I made a futile attempt to listen to the rest of my patient's reports, cocking my head in a seemingly intelligent pose. But basically they were all the same gibberish.

As report ended, the crowd began to disperse into a flurry of self-directed activity. I followed a knowing crowd to the linen room and watched as one LPN, Molly, expertly stacked her linens for each room on a cart. Blanket, bedspread, sheet, draw-sheet, pull sheet, sheet, pillowcase, towel, towel, washcloth, repeat. When she got to five sets, she loaded the stack in her arms and left. When it was my turn, I gathered what was left of the linens and delivered them to my rooms, walking as quietly as I could so as not to wake up any of my patients. I didn't want them asking me any questions.

I snuck back to the nurses' station that by this time was vacant with the exception of a secretary who had just arrived and was casually unpacking her lunch and purse at her desk.

"Hi, I'm Rose," she said, smiling. "You're our new grad aren't you? I remember seeing you when you went on tour the other day. How's your first day going?"

"Fine, I guess. I'm a little overwhelmed right now."

"Oh you'll do fine. It takes awhile, but they all start out that way. If you need anything, let me know."

"Thanks."

I needed that. I've always found homage and security with a mom figure in reach.

I spotted the patient information kardex on the desk. Feeling like I had no right to be anywhere near it, I half-opened it to Mr. Sabatini's record. Under "Doctor" it had neatly listed "DMSV". Under "Diagnosis", it had "Revision of CABG". Mrs. Smythe's kardex was no better, but at least now I knew "TAHBSO" was a surgery. But what kind? Carol appeared at my side with a steaming cup of coffee in her hand.

"Are you okay?" she asked.

Was the loss of all coloring from my face that obvious? I had been the top student in my nursing baccalaureate class and yet here I stood, looking at a gal who had "only a hospital diploma" to her name and SHE knew every disease and doctor by the first letter only AND spoke lab values like she understood them. It was at that moment that I realized how little I really knew and I really hated the fact that I was going to have to admit it. Hospital-based diploma student nurses generally had more opportunities to practice their skills with actual patients since the hospitals unofficially used them to help staff their floors. A Baccalaureate nursing program provides a traditional college experience with one to two clinical days weekly over the four years. As a result, the diploma nurses were more technically competent immediate upon graduation. Some of the diploma nurses resented the baccalaureate graduates because they were quickly advanced to management and leadership roles.

I took a deep breath and said, "I haven't the foggiest idea what is wrong with my patients. What is a TAHBSO?" I braced myself for the expected fall out.

"I can't believe they didn't teach you that in nursing school. It stands for Total Abdominal Hysterectomy with a Bilateral Salpinooopherectomy."

"OH", I said, as all kinds of lights switched on in my head.

My patient was post-op from a removal of the uterus, tubes and ovaries. I knew how to care for that. Carol patiently explained all the abbreviations to me, like a beacon of light in a fog leading a ship safe to port. Armed with new knowledge, I confidently headed back towards my first room. Vital signs were first. "Okay, I can do that," I told myself.

Twenty minutes later I had finally found the blood pressure cuff and the electronic thermometer. By that time, three of my patients' lights had gone on. I suddenly felt like a waitress again, in the middle of a lunchtime rush with everyone asking for separate checks. Looking nervously at my watch, I headed into Room 15.

"Nurse, I need the bedpan. I've had my light on for twenty minutes. Where is everybody?"

I politely explained that I was her nurse and would be glad to assist her onto the bedpan. I opened the bedside stand, standard hospital furniture, but found only a wash basin and a soiled nighty. I went to the bathroom and looked around. No bedpan. Desperate, I headed down the hall to the clean utility room where I had remembered seeing some bedpans stored during my orientation tour. I grabbed one and sped back to Room 15.

As I pulled back the sheet to place the patient on the bedpan, I found Mrs. Smythe's bedpan lying next to her already.

"I like it close," she said smiling at me.

I put the extra bedpan in the chair and proceeded to attempt to get this relatively obese woman onto the pan. Mrs. Smythe managed to roll her upper body by grasping the side rail, but her voluminous thighs and buttocks hadn't budged. I can do this, I thought. With a heave ho, I took her right hip and gave it a good push. It was like trying to hold a bowl of jello back with one hand. While still holding her overflowing hip with one hand, I attempted to position the bedpan under her, pushing hard with the other hand. I pulled her back over top of it. I thought.

"I don't think I'm on it nurse. Ewwww, I gotta go..."

"Hold on, I'll try again."

"Hurry."

We repeated the laborious procedure again, this time gaining enough ground so that once she had been rolled over flat, the bedpan disappeared from view. One could only guess where it actually was positioned.

"Go for it," I said, praying.

"Put my head up," she demanded.

I looked for the electric bed controls to no avail. Mrs. Smythe impatiently pointed to the crank at the foot of the bed. So much for a therapeutic relationship with this patient, I thought. I cranked her to a height she found satisfactory and pulled her curtain closed just as Leah came grumbling in the door.

"If you are in here, turn off the damn light."

"I'm sorry." She watched me as I went to the call light on the wall and pressed the wrong button.

"It's the other one."

"Oh, everything is so different here from what I was used to in school," attempting to save some face.

"Uhh huh. I put your other patients on the bedpan, but I don't have time to get them off. I'm going on break." She left the room.

I hadn't even left the room before Mrs. Smythe called out from behind the curtain, "I'm done Nurse."

I gathered some tissue, as though it was possible for me to even find what to wipe, and began to turn her to her left side again. So did the bedpan. It had formed a tight suction to her buttocks in just those brief moments, and I had to pry it with my ungloved finger to break the suction. Back then, gloves were expensive and only made available for sterile procedures, never for routine hygiene no matter how disgusting the clean up. That's what hand washing was for. The bedpan gave way with a potentially splashing jolt. Ahh success, I thought, no splash. Removing the bedpan, I prepared to examine the urine for color, odor, and amount as I was taught. Unfortunately, the bedpan was empty. My thoughts were interrupted.

"Nurse, I feel wet."

I soon discovered that an out of sight bedpan does not insure proper placement. I gathered the necessary materials, and with lots of prodding, pushing, and poking, I was able to successfully change and clean Mrs. Smythe up. Sweat poured from my brow, but I stood back knowing that I had done the job well. I checked my watch. This had only taken thirty minutes. It was after 8:30 a.m. I had still not checked any of my other patients. My vital signs were not finished. Thank God we had a medication nurse or I would have lost my license before I received it in the mail.

Calla, a veteran RN, entered with some medication for Mrs. Smythe. I moved to the patient with the window view bed and quickly took a set of vital signs, carefully recording each value as I got it. Mrs. Gomez asked for her basin saying she preferred bathing herself before breakfast. Delighted, I took her basin to the bathroom and filled it with warm water. As I left Mrs. Gomez,

Mrs. Smythe called out.

"Nurse, before you go. I need the bedpan again."

My mouth resounded with "Sure", but my heart sank into my shoes. I got her bedpan out again and asked her, once again, to go on her side. Just then, Calla walked past with Mrs. Gomez's medications.

"I'll help you in a second," she said. "Mrs. Smythe is impossible to do by yourself."

No kidding I thought. I just hoped Mrs. Smythe wouldn't embarrass me by telling Calla what had happened already this morning. Calla helped to boost Mrs. Smythe way over on her side by using the pull sheet and pulling, not pushing, towards herself. She positioned the bedpan centered over her buttocks, then telling me to push down firmly on the bedpan, she rolled her over again. Once over, she peeked between her legs to see if the pan was in the right spot. "Go for it!" we said. I could have kissed Calla right there and then.

Calla told Mrs. Smythe that it was my very first day and that they were glad to have another body to rotate to nights. Mrs. Smythe smiled and said, "She's going to make a good nurse...someday."

Leah stopped by to tell me that she had taken my patients off their bedpans for me and that her break was shortened because of it. I thanked her profusely, unaware at the time that it was her job that day to help answer all of the lights. I eventually got my vital signs done, despite having to wait another thirty minutes to take the temperatures since most of my patients had started to eat breakfast, which would have invalidated the reading.

I then set-up the other patients that could bathe themselves then returned to bathe Mrs. Smythe. Patients with that much body surface area should really count for two people. Her bath took me over an hour, so by the time I got back to my other patients to finish their backs or hard to reach areas, most had given up waiting and had already gotten dressed.

Doctors came in and out asking me questions, which I rarely knew the answer to. My answer for the day was consistently, "It's my first day here, I don't know anything." One doctor responded by introducing himself and welcoming me. The others generally looked aggravated and asked, "Then who does?"

I actually did the noon vital signs at noon, though most of the patients wanted to know why I was doing it again so soon. Carol came and made me take a lunch break at 12:30. So I did the dressings scheduled for the morning after lunch. All my patients' bed-sheets were changed by 2:30. I even had a chance to sit and talk with my pre-operative patient, Mr. Sabatini, about his "cabbage", an open heart surgery that he was really worried about.

Now all I had to do was chart everything I had done all day. We used longhand narrative notes and had to reconstruct each patient's day on an hour by hour basis. By 3:30, I had pretty much had it.

Rose watched as I put my last chart in the rack. "You made it. I told you everything would be fine. Two weeks from now, it will be simple!"

My feet were sore, my legs ached, my make-up had long since worn off, my armpits had overpowered the deodorant, and my pen had leaked all over my right hand. I was not a foreigner to labor, having worked my way through college as a waitress in an ice cream restaurant. But as I reached my hands into my pockets and found them totally devoid of tips, I wasn't sure what the rewards of this job would be, let alone what kind of profession I had really gotten myself into.

I felt as though I had left dozens of things undone. Mrs. Smythe's hair needed to be washed. I hadn't done my other patient's backs. My morning vital signs had been two hours late. I needed three more hours between 8 and 9 a.m. to do my job the way I thought it should be done.

Throughout the day, I had vacillated between anger and disappointment at my college program for sending me out with theories, not experiences; expecting me to apply what we learned on the run. I thought back to my lazy learning lab teachers, whose idea of teaching skills was to turn on a movie and give us free reign to practice the skills after class on our own, unsupervised. The time-consuming skill performance validations were outdated they said. So here I was, green on the vine, plucked and tossed into the fray, stuffed full of whys and science, but with few "how to" memories to rely on.

I found my coat and headed off the floor. Passing Mr. Sabatini in the hallway, he stopped me and held my arm. "Thanks

for listening today. Nobody else had the time."
Neither did I Mr. Sabatini. Neither did I.

"If the axe is dull and it's edge unsharpened, more strength is needed but skill will bring success."

Ecclesiastes 10:10

2

The Cath Queen

Several months had gone by and Rose's prediction had come to pass. Having five or six patients became routine and I became organized enough to get backs washed and massaged, feet soaked and skin lubed. I could even hear blood pressures with faint and erratic sounds and feel pulses with rates that ran faster than the average person's counting speed. My dressings were done on time and I had even survived my first enema, thanks to the instructions on the side of the box. Despite that, my minimal clinical experience from school continued to haunt me.

Mrs. Baxter was a 74 year old woman admitted for senile dementia. She had multiple medical problems, not the least of which was urinary retention and incontinence. The doctor ordered her to be catheterized, a procedure that requires placing a tube into the urethra to drain urine. In nursing classes, we practiced catheterization technique on mannequins that had no pubic hair and 3 distinct holes, each the size of dimes. The opportunity to catheterize a real patient in a clinical was based on luck, not design. I had been a lucky one, replacing a catheter on a patient whose urethral opening was the size of our mannequins, thanks to years of pulling hers out with the 30 cc, golf ball size balloon inflated.

"Do you feel comfortable catheterizing Mrs. Baxter by yourself?" Carol asked.

Based on prior experiences, I felt very confident in this area. "No problem."

I expertly prepared all of my materials and explained the intended procedure to my patient.

"Who are you?"

"I'm your nurse, Karen, Mrs. Baxter. I was the one who gave you your bath this morning."

"Oh, I remember you Kathy."

"The doctor wants you to have a tube to empty your urine."

"I have no urine."

"No, the doctor wants you to have a tube put into your bladder to empty the urine that's in there."

"Okay, let's go to the doctor," Mrs. Baxter said as she started to get out of bed.

"No Mrs. Baxter. We don't have to go anywhere right now."

"I'm going to the doctor."

"The doctor's busy right now. I'm going to have to catheterize you."

"Why didn't you say so?"

"Okay. I'm going to need you to lie back and relax."

"Okay. But I have no urine."

"Mrs. Baxter, I'm ready to catheterize you now."

"Who are you?"

I didn't try to explain again. Fortunately, Mrs. Baxter was relatively compliant with instructions, despite her otherwise apparent confusion. I spread her legs, positioned my light and meticulously put on my sterile gloves. Spreading her labia per procedure, I began cleansing her perineal area. I could see her clitoral hood and vagina clearly, but the dime-size urethral opening I expected to see between them was nowhere in sight. I cleansed with my last wipe, hoping that magically, the urethral opening would appear, but it didn't. I used my sterile hand to look around a little out of desperation.

"What are you doing down there?" asked the voice from the other end of the bed.

"I'm getting ready to catheterize you Mrs. Baxter."

"Oh."

"I'm sorry if it hurts."

"It doesn't hurt."

Realizing the need to get on with this procedure, I poked my catheter at a speck that I hoped would be her urethral opening. No opening there, just a speck. I poked under the clitoral hood. Nothing. My grasp on her labia loosened and I could feel the catheter enter. Yes. I gently pushed the catheter in further, further. Check the tubing, no sign of urine yet. Further, further until I spotted the tip of the catheter coming back at me. That is something that happens when the catheter is inadvertently placed in the vagina. Problem was, now it was contaminated and having no extra catheter or gloves, I would need to get an entirely new set up from the supply room.

I snuck out of the room, walking casually past the nurses' station to the supply room to get another kit. The staff had already had a field day mocking me for so many things I had not ever done in my clinical training, that I REALLY wanted to do this one on my own. I hid the catheterization kit from view as I retreated back to Mrs. Baxter's room, with renewed expectations. I could do this.

I started from scratch looking again very carefully for some missed dimple or divot that just might be the urethral opening. And after carefully selecting my new approach, I repeated the earlier "vaginal" catheterization.

"Are you done yet?" asked the woman behind the drapes.

"No, Mrs. Baxter," covering her private area again, "I'll be back in a minute."

My patient's personal comfort and dignity has always come above my own, so I sought out my preceptor Carol and admitted shamefully, that I had tried twice, but hadn't been able to successfully catheterize Mrs. Baxter.

"Don't worry, some of them are really hard to find...it's not like the mannequin is it?"

"Not at all."

Unfortunately for Mrs. Baxter, Carol was unsuccessful as well. Outwardly I expressed a sincere concern for the difficult nature of this procedure. Inside, I said, "Yes! It's not just me!"

Carol looked at me very seriously and said, "Karen, this is a job for the Cath Queen."

The Cath Queen of our unit was a LPN named Ellen who was efficient and reliable. LPN's are Licensed Practical Nurses that undergo one year of training focusing primarily on skills and procedures. They receive only a brief overview of medical knowledge, whereas RN's (Registered Nurses) have either a two year (Associate's degree), three year (Hospital diploma), or four year (Baccalaureate degree) program. The RN program adds the study of disease processes and management, along with the assessment and treatment of patient's across the wellness to illness spectrum for all developmental stages of life. In addition to direct patient care, RN's are prepared to provide health education, counseling, and function independently in community settings. Advanced practice nurses (Nurse Practitioners) at the master's level are licensed to diagnose and treat acute and chronic illness and prescribe medications. Doctoral level nurses are the researchers, educators, and/or clinical experts in their fields of specialty. While all carry the basic title of "nurse", there are huge educational differences among them.

Ellen loved her Cath Queen title, and was eager to flaunt her talent amongst the RN's with any elusive urethra. Ellen walked in, joked with Mrs. Baxter about how a real nurse would fix her up. She put on her gloves with a loud snap. She took the woman's droopy perineal area and with one swift tug towards her abdomen, had created an entirely different viewing area. The dimple sized urethra suddenly became visible as she quickly popped the catheter in to produce a rapid outpouring of urine.

"Anytime, girls!" she said as she tossed her gloves into the discard pile on the bed and then pranced out the door. I cleaned Mrs. Baxter up and reminded her that she had a tube in her now so that she didn't need to urinate in the bedpan anymore.

Mrs. Baxter winked and said, "Sweetie, I never used the bedpan anyway. Are we going to the Doctor now?"

"Listen to advice and accept instruction and in the end you will be wise."

Proverbs 19:20

3

Welcome to Nights

I had no idea how to prepare to work a night shift. Should I bring food? Should I nap before I leave? Should I leave my contacts in? No one in my family had ever worked nights before, so they were of little help. It felt odd saying good-bye as they donned their jammies and drank their night caps.

As I walked into the building from the closest parking spot I had ever gotten at a hospital, I could hear the stillness of the night settling in. My body, hearing nature's whispers, asked me how much longer before we too went to bed.

The hospital lobby was empty with the exception of one half-alert security guard using a pillar as a leaning post. He nodded vaguely at my passing. The lights in the patient hallways were dim as I approached the now familiar nurses' station.

I recognized most of the women in the station. The evening staff who I had passed report to at 3 p.m. for the past six months appeared less fresh than usual. They were busy charting and making after work plans. The night staff was made up of mostly stoic older women. From their pallor, I suspected most slept during the daylight hours. The night shift's businesslike approach contrasted severely against the evening gang's casual gaiety and they began to appear restless for the report to begin and the confusion to dissipate.

Soon the report was over and the evening shift was on their way. Their echoes of laughter filtered down the hallway, then abruptly stopped, sealed behind the closed elevator doors. I was alone with these strange women, and as the only RN on duty, I was in charge and feeling entirely like a fish out of water.

My cohort group of 21 year old peers was likely hanging out enjoying themselves at some bar, as I assumed full responsibility on my RN license for the lives of every patient on the ward. I will never forget the chills in my spine the first time I saw the words,

"K. Smith RN notified" on a chart. Being in charge is not for the faint of heart. Your eyes, ears, and brain are required to be on high alert the entire time, regardless of the shift you are on.

The staff was quick to tell me just what I could and could not expect of them. The two aides headed down the hall to the break-room and the LPN went off the check the post-ops because that was "what she always did." I began a mix of clerical and managerial chores then headed out to make rounds and give my midnight medications. The aides appeared again at some point to tell me what they planned to do next and to ask me if I wanted anything from the cafeteria.

I quickly learned that on a quiet night, the most challenging responsibility of the night staff was to stay awake and alert. Most full-time night staff met this challenge by eating. Some staff ate continuously; others ate one larger meal after 3 a.m. Some staff called this "dinner"; others called it "breakfast". The inevitable smorgasbord varied from night to night, and always seemed to prevent the nods.

Finding nighttime eating personally disruptive, I selected to do busywork instead. Floors traditionally assign a multitude of paperwork and chart checking chores to the night staff. I found these beneficial to get to the 3 a.m. mark, but on that first quiet night I fell sound asleep in the chart rack somewhere between 3 and 4. Thereafter, I learned to get up and take rounds whenever the nods came on.

That first night I was introduced to the syndrome of "Butt Inertia." This would develop when a patient call light would go on after a 1-2 hour period of silence. Regardless of how much energy you generally had, or how bored you thought you had become, the sudden interruption to peace was seldom welcomed. The staff would barter their last candy bar to avoid moving, once butt inertia had set in.

Another oddity of nights was the unique communication system. To understand it, first you must remember that you are a walking zombie trying to function at peak intelligence. Second of all, the staff you think you are communicating with are also walking zombies. Most importantly, it's dark. Ears don't work as well in dim light.

"Diane, what did Mr. Song's dressing look like?"

"I thought you said you'd check it."

"I did Mr. Thompson's dressing."

"So did I, I wondered why there was no drainage on it."

Twenty minutes later. "So how was Mr. Song's dressing?"

"I thought you were going to check it." etc. etc. Eventually, someone checked Mr. Song's dressing.

Once that first night began to get busier, I gained a new perspective of this nocturnal staff. Lights on both ends of the hall flickered on like a busy switchboard, with each patient's call probably awakening the next. The night staff women worked quickly and efficiently in teams, moving from one room to the next, leaving only satisfied and comfortable patients in their wake. They rolled patients to new sides, changed wet linen or dressings, and walked patients to the bathroom.

It was apparent that these women flourished in this atmosphere of freedom from supervision. They devised creative solutions for a multitude of patient problems, like unique ways to secure IV's or hold ice bags to odd body parts. Night nurses learned to trust their instincts and quickly distinguished significant signs and symptoms from the insignificant. That was especially important at night when in the dim light a dying patient could be mistaken for a sleeping patient. Unlike the day shift, where nurses are surrounded by others with experience, on the night shift, autonomy was induced. Self reliance was a necessity.

My first night, I hadn't quite developed those skills.

"Dr. Abbott, this is Karen Smith, Charge Nurse on 5 North at Main Hospital."

"What time is it?"

"It's 4:30 a.m."

"You've got to be kidding. I don't even have any patients on 5."

"Mrs. Benjamin, post-op appendectomy from yesterday."

"Okay, okay, this better be good."

"Mrs. Benjamin's temperature is 101.2 rectally and the Tylenol order I have is for pain only."

"You woke me at 4:30 to ask me for a lousy Tylenol rewrite? Where's the damn resident?"

"I'm sorry Dr. Abbott, but the resident has been tied up for hours."

Dr. Abbott gave me the order and slammed down the phone.

Betty, the LPN, overheard my end of the conversation. "Not real happy about the call, huh?"

"It wasn't like I had any choice," I responded.

"You're the charge," she replied with emphasis on the "you're" accompanied by a judgmental brow raise as she returned to her charting.

Dr. Abbott arrived on the floor around 6:30 that morning. As I neared the station, I overheard him talking to Betty.

"Do you know what idiot nurse called me at 3:15 this morning for a Tylenol order?" Dr. Abbott's voice was quite expressive.

"That was Karen."

"Where is she? I have a few choice words for her."

"She's our new grad. Her first time on nights. Go easy on her."

I had wisely chosen to remain out of sight.

Dr. Abbott gathered his gear. "I've got to get to the OR. Get her straightened out, or I will."

"Sure, Doc," Betty replied in a non-confrontational tone. "Have a good day."

"Right."

I pretended to read my clipboard as Dr. Abbott exited the station. As he passed me, he glanced knowingly, with a millisecond of hesitation in his step. I looked up, visibly devoid of armor, and gave him my best smile, effectively melting his fury. With a sympathetic glance, he headed out to save some more lives.

I walked into the station. "I heard him, Betty. You don't have to tell me."

"He's really a pretty nice guy. You can trust him to write whatever orders you need in the morning. He always stops by before surgery."

"Thanks. I'm still learning. What else did I screw up?"

"Nothing. You did real good tonight," Betty said reassuringly. "Now don't you worry about him. Cute young nurses can do no harm."

Great, just what I needed to know. He thought I was a cute, lousy nurse!

Report went well and soon I found myself heading home. I drove without the radio on, alone with my thoughts, analyzing my performance, and planning what to do differently next time. Pretty soon I found myself being gradually lulled to sleep by the hum of the engine.

Somewhere a voice inside said, "NOT YET!" and I shook myself awake. I opened the car windows wide to the chilly morning air and blared the radio as loud as my ears would tolerate. The last few miles I had to slap my arms and thighs and stamp my non-driving foot to prevent my lapse into unconsciousness. I passed my rested parents on the way to my room. "You look awful!" Mom said.

Welcome to nights.

***"Even youths grow tired and weary,
and young men stumble and fall; but those who hope in
the Lord will renew their strength.
They will soar on wings like eagles; they will run and
not grow weary, they will walk and not be faint."***

Isaiah 40:29-31

4

The Night From Hell

Ask any emergency room, labor and delivery, or night nurse and they will all tell you the same thing. Try not to work the night of a full moon. Sociologists won't back us up statistically, but remember, they work numbers, not nights.

"Full moon tonight, wasn't it pretty?" I said politely. Even though I had worked many weeks of nights by now, as a day shift floater, I was still considered a foreigner to the night staff so I tried to stay on neutral topics.

"Don't mention it. Last full moon I worked, this place went nuts," Annabelle offered.

"What do you mean?"

"Don't scare her Annabelle. There have been plenty of quiet full moons too and you know it. You is just superstitious." Lillie was a big black gal with a heavy Southern accent.

"Remember that Mr. Peters? He damn near got himself killed." Annabelle turned and spoke quietly to me. "The police found him stark naked in the tennis court across the street. No one even knew he had left."

"Annabelle, Mr. Peters did that all the time. That was just a coincidence."

"Yeah, well when you start finding patients lying on the floor, don't call me to help you."

"Oh, stop!" Lillie shook her head.

By 2 a.m., almost snooze-time, Annabelle had relaxed. It looked like a normal night after all. I took off on rounds with my trusty flashlight. All quiet on the North wing. Heading to the South wing, I entered Mr. Jones room and noticed he wasn't in his bed. Mr. Jones was an elderly gentleman in for diagnostic tests. I checked the bathroom. "Mr. Jones?" Empty. I scanned my flashlight around, half-expecting him to jump out of the closet and scare me. But there he was, just sitting on the window side of the bed, on the floor, quiet as a mouse. I called out into the hallway for help then moved to his side.

"Mr. Jones, are you okay?"

"Sure."

"What are you doing down here on the floor?"

"I sat down."

"But why were you getting out of bed?"

"Well, you see, I was on my way to the bank to make a deposit, but I got tired, so I sat down."

"Mr. Jones, you're in the hospital. I'm your nurse."

"Oops, I forgot."

The resident on duty had to be called to check Mr. Jones. One hour and four calls later, the harried looking resident finally arrived. We weren't the only ones having a crazy night. The emergency room was filled and ICU had two patients "going bad." By that time, Mr. Jones was sound asleep and less than pleased to be awaked for this perfunctory exam. The resident ordered X-rays to cover himself, even though there were no obvious signs of injury. When the X-ray department arrived with their portable machine, once again Mr. Jones had just drifted off to sleep. The normally timid Mr. Jones became irate. He allowed the X-ray but his angry responses woke all the neighboring patients initiating a flurry of call lights and medication requests that spread like a wave down the entire hall.

By the time the dust settled from the paperwork that the incident had generated, it was already time to make rounds again. As I opened the door of one of my post-op prostate resection patients, I was startled to find him standing just inside his doorway with the front of his gown stained with blood.

"What the heck?" I flipped on the light to see blood everywhere, sprayed all over the walls, floors, and even the other patient's bed. It looked like a crime scene with only the chalk body outline and yellow police tape missing. It didn't take long to figure out what had happened.

This gentleman belonged in the bed near the window. His "foley" urine catheter bag was still properly attached to the side of his bed. The patient had felt the urge to use the bathroom, which was located a good twenty feet away by the door. His catheter had the capability of stretching about nine feet under test conditions. Once stretched beyond the limit, the catheter had pulled out like a cork and sprayed his bloody urine everywhere. Amazingly, he had no pain, nor did he really comprehend what had happened, despite the fact that he was normally a totally coherent, active, sixty year old man.

The resident was not pleased to have to return again so soon. His beeper went off four times while he reinserted a new catheter. When he was done, the sleep deprived resident scratched a barely legible note in the chart, stole one of Annabelle's cupcakes with a sheepish grin, then bolted down the hallway and disappeared into the stairwell. I returned to the room to clean up.

On the way out of the room, I noticed that his roommate, another post-op prostate resection, had blood all over his freshly changed sheets. At first, I thought it was from his roommate. At closer evaluation, I realized that it was because his IV had been pulled out and had made quite a mess. He swore it came out accidentally, despite the fact that I found the IV needle hurled across the room and the tape carefully removed, one piece at a time and stuck to the bed-sheets. I restarted his IV, changed the bloody linen and turned out the light to the room. As I left, I didn't bother to pull out my flashlight. The rays of the large white moon already brightened the room.

Although some night shifts seem like they'll never end, by 6 a.m., I had begun to play beat the clock. With a tremendous effort, I managed to get the important stuff done, like patient care, medications, and vital documentation. The staff had worked very hard that night and I was sure to let them know how wonderful they had all been through this difficult and busy shift. We took turns offering accolades to each other. I was still feeling great about myself when I gave an enthusiastic report on what had been an exciting, challenging night. The response from the groggy pre-coffee day shift was nevertheless a disappointment.

"Did you run today's lab slips?"

"Where are the IV stock requisitions?"

"I see the anesthesia consent wasn't signed yet for the pre-op for this morning."

As I looked around at the 6 RN's, 2 LPN's, 2 Nurses Aides and the secretary who had come on duty to replace the 1 RN, 1

LPN and 2 Aides who had just put in a night from hell, my face likely assumed that same stoic mask I had often seen on women of the night shift. I was incredulous of the day shifts' naivety of the horrendous night we had just survived.

The crisp air of winter stung my face as I left the hospital that morning. I looked up at the early morning sky, my eyes drawn to the remnant gleam of the full moon, laughing at me as it faded away behind some wispy clouds.

"He leads me beside the still waters.
He restores my soul."

Psalm 23:2-3

5

When you shouldn't hear, "Oops!"

"You're back. Last time we saw you it was a full moon."

"Not tonight, thank goodness. I could use a quiet night. What's in your goodie bag tonight Annabelle?"

"Homemade soup and biscuits. Decided I would cook for the family tonight for a change."

"What's the occasion?" Lillie interrupted. "It isn't Christmas yet Annabelle!"

"Oh stop it you hear or I'll make you do Room 5 by yourself."

Conversations were predictably light. Lots of teasing, lots of jokes. In medicine, it's survival. It is part escape from and part denial of the real life tragedies we align ourselves with on a day to day basis. Lillie and Annabelle were still exchanging barbs as they headed out to start their care.

It was almost 2 a.m. when Annabelle rushed into the nurses' station. Her voice was firm and fast.

"Karen, I think you better check Mrs. Campbell." We ran back down the hall, the others followed.

Mrs. Campbell was not breathing and from her stiffened extremities, pallor, dropped jaw, and staring eyes, an experienced nurse would have immediately recognized that this woman had been dead for some time. Mrs. Campbell was the first patient to die while I was in charge. The staff looked at me, awaiting orders.

"Does anybody know if she's a code or not?" I asked quickly moving her to CPR position. The LPN stood back against the wall. "She's 87 years old. Let her go."

If I had been watching this happen on a movie, I would have known exactly what to do and would have agreed with my LPN. But faced with the decision myself, all I could think of was policies, procedures and legalities. If Mrs. Campbell was not a "no code", we would code her. I instructed the others to begin CPR while I ran to the nurses' station to check the kardex. The line on the kardex next to "Code Status" was blank and I didn't see anything else written so I pushed the red button on the wall and the code alarm sounded.

"CODE BLUE 5 NORTH," crackled on the PA system, breaking the silence.

People descended upon the unit in droves. Respiratory therapy, ICU nurses, EKG technicians, the resident on duty, and the house supervisors. I hadn't even realized how many other employees were in the building! But within minutes, these experienced staff reemerged from the patient's room and regrouped in the nurses' station.

"Who the hell called a code on her?"

"She's probably been dead for hours!"

"They don't need resuscitation, they need a resurrection!"

"I'd start CPR, but I can't get her flat enough." Laughter ensued.

I felt really stupid and embarrassed. Unfortunately, there was nowhere for me to hide. The Nurse Supervisor entered the station with a scornful look. I braced myself for the worst.

"Why was this code called?" she asked.

"I really wasn't sure what to do," I replied sheepishly. "She wasn't a no code."

The supervisor brushed past me and looked through the nursing kardex. "What does this say here?"

Right on the top of the front of the kardex, in red, were the words, "No code". My mouth dropped open as I looked at the neatly, albeit small, but undeniably clear message on the kardex.

"I didn't see it. Honest I looked. It was blank on the section next to Code Status."

She looked but found little merit to my words.

"This is very costly to the hospital. You have to be more careful in the future."

"Yes maam." There was nothing more to say. At least I wasn't fired.

Years later, when I was the expert ICU nurse responding to a code on another med-surg unit, an inexperienced nurse had called a code on a man with terminal cancer. I overheard the technician comfort the embarrassed nurse by saying, "That's okay. This isn't so bad. I responded to a code once that a new nurse had called when the patient had so much rigor mortis already we couldn't even straighten her out on the board!"

That time I joined in with the laughter, grateful I wasn't recognized.

Once the unit had cleared that fateful night, I went through the kardex carefully and marked the NO CODE patients very clearly several times on each kardex. Then I listed them on my charge report sheet. I went upon my duties with renewed diligence, determined to not make any other mistakes that night.

As the only RN on the floor, I had sole responsibility for all the intravenous solutions (IV's). Before mechanical pumps were used so extensively, nurses had to calculate the number of drops per minute of an IV solution and then manually adjust the flow rate every hour. In order to do that, the nurse would count the drops as they fell, then speed or slow the rate using a roller clamp device on the tubing. If an IV needle were leaning against the inside of a vein, moving the arm might make a difference in how fast the solution would flow. Nurses referred to this IV as "positional." Unfortunately, you wouldn't know an IV was positional until the patient moved it.

Ida Ryan was an 83 year old woman admitted because of dehydration. She had a history of congestive heart failure, which meant that her heart was not working effectively as a pump, making it harder to move blood through her body. Naturally, IV fluids had to be given carefully since it isn't safe to overload an already weak pump.

All night, Ida had slept soundly, and her IV, running at a slow 50 cc per hour was right on schedule at each hourly check. During 0600 rounds, I hung a new IV, then returned to the nurses' station to finish my paperwork before shift change report.

Mandy, an extremely efficient staff RN arrived early and made her IV rounds before she had even put her coat away. "Do you have Mrs. Ryan's next IV ready? It's almost empty."

"You're kidding aren't you?" I asked, but she looked serious. I jumped from my seat and dashed into the room. Ida, still sleeping, had rolled over in bed, and the IV had emptied rapidly into her arm. 950 cc in about thirty minutes. That was enough to provide a deadly challenge to a weak heart. I slowed her IV to a near trickle, cranked the head of her bed up and instructed my aide, who appeared ready for action to hunt down the blood pressure cuff.

The angels were with Ida that night. She was fine, thanks only to her pre-existing dehydration and healthy kidneys. I was told she urinated all morning long but couldn't understand why. We didn't always tell patients about the near misses back then.

My night staff made polite comments of support to me as they left that morning, but I knew that this night had been a disaster. Although no one was harmed, I had still made two blaring errors, one potentially serious. I had provided the anti-baccalaureates with fresh juicy ammunition and felt I had destroyed my credibility as a potentially efficient charge nurse.

There was no chance of falling asleep that morning on the drive home in the car as I relived my errors as though watching a film loop. I chastised myself as though total perfection in nursing was within my grasp. Determined to never let mistakes like these happen again, I revised my priorities. I planned to watch the others closely, learn from them and follow their lead of making policy and routines my priority.

***"I am determined to be wise, but this is beyond me.
Whatever wisdom may be,
it is far off and most profound.
Who can discover it?
So I turned my mind to understand,
to investigate and to search out wisdom
and the scheme of things..."***

Ecclesiastes 7:23-5

6

Priorities

After several more months, the "Miss Baccalaureate" jokes had slowed to a trickle; in fact, the staff was encouraged by my progress under their tutelage. By hospital standards, I had become a "good" nurse. My paperwork was always complete and my IV's were running on time. I enjoyed being in charge again and found the pressure invigorating. I was even helping to orient another new graduate. It was with renewed confidence that I made my rounds one quiet night shift.

Mrs. Moore was 28, had three young children under the age of six and was dying of ovarian cancer. Her eyes and cheeks were sunken as her skin clung to its' bony structure, her frail petite frame overwhelmed by the massive hospital bed. She was in constant pain and the morphine injections were no longer providing adequate relief. Many of our patients died in pain back then, before the days of morphine drips. Mrs. Moore was not an exception.

She was awake when I entered her room on tiptoes with my tiny flashlight. I could see her eyes follow me as I entered the room, her body too weak to move. She asked me, through parched lips, "Could I have my next pain shot?"

I knew that it wasn't time yet without even checking, but I told her, "I'll sneak it to you a half hour early."

I put some lubricant on her lips and adjusted her sheets knowing that legally, that was all I could offer at this time.

I continued on with my rounds and got lost in my "important busy work" at the desk. A while later, I got one of those funny feelings, the kind nurses learn not to ignore. So I took rounds again. When I got to Mrs. Moore, she was laying on her side, where I had left her, hands clenched tightly to the side rails with her eyes staring wild eyed into space. She was dead.

While I dotted the i's and crossed the t's that night, Mrs.

Moore died in pain, alone and scared in the dark. I had been so proud of my managerial skills, as I played "super Charge Nurse", that I had forgotten to nurse.

Perhaps I was more comforting to Mr. Moore when he came to the hospital that night, but he was probably too numb to notice. It was a sad way to learn my lesson on real priorities.

When I returned to the day shift I was assigned to Mrs. Webster, a classy lady in her fifties, with newly diagnosed diabetes who was as eager to learn about her disease as I was to teach her. Each day she got progressively more confident that she would be able to manage this complex condition herself at home. Getting to know her, and hearing about her family, full grown children, loving husband and her new career goals, I had little doubt that Mrs. Webster would be successful.

On Friday, the day Mrs. Webster was to be discharged, I took report.

"What time is Mrs. Webster due to leave?" I asked in anticipation of the report.

"She's not leaving today," the night nurse informed me.

"Why not?" I asked, inwardly making plans to take on the doctors for the unnecessary delays.

"Apparently it isn't routine diabetes like they thought. She has pancreatic cancer and it's inoperable. They told her on evenings."

"Not Mrs. Webster," my mouth dropping open.

"I don't know her," the night nurse replied nonchalantly. She continued on with report about how Mrs. Webster still needed to continue with the diabetic teaching plan as well as other tangible components of her medical needs. Not a word was said about her emotional state or needs.

When I entered the room after report, Mrs. Webster, obviously awake for hours, forced a cheery smile and asked me how I was doing, pointedly keeping the conversation light and centered away from her. It was in character for her to not want to burden another with her personal tragedy. I played along though my insides ached from fighting back tears. I wanted to say so much more, like how unfair it was for someone so kind to be given such a bad deal. But I knew I didn't have the time right now to open up a wound that big.

"How many patients do you have today?" Mrs. Webster asked.

She looked like she wanted to talk and what she was really asking was, "How much time do you have for me?" Her world was collapsing but she didn't want to interfere with my busy morning assignment, so instead she put up the facade of normalcy. I promised Mrs. Webster that I would stop back for a chat as soon as I could.

All morning long, it was as though I was tied to a heavy rope that tugged at me in the direction of Mrs. Webster's room. Each unexpected additional chore only frustrated my attempts to get back to her. Finally, it was lunchtime. I stood next to my open locker, inhaled my sandwich, and then snuck back into Mrs. Webster's room, to avoid being seen by my other patients. I pulled a chair up close to her bed and sat down.

"Now," I said pausing to sigh as though catching my breath. I looked deeply into Mrs. Webster's eyes. "How are you really doing?"

"I'm so glad you came in," Mrs. Webster breathed deeply. "I can't believe this is really happening."

"Neither can I. It's not fair."

"You know, when they first told me I had diabetes I was in shock. I had been really upset those first couple of days, but you helped me through them. I was really getting the hang of the diet and the shots, thanks to you. It's kinda funny, but I had been angry that I was going to have to live with a chronic disease." She stopped and half laughed as she looked off into space, lost in her own thoughts. "Now I wish I could live with a chronic disease."

I reached up for her hand. We squeezed hands tightly and when our eyes met, we were both filling with tears.

"I'm going to be here for you," I said quietly.

The conversation lightened as Mrs. Webster found a way to get me to tell a story that would cheer her up. Just then, the day supervisor burst into the room, appalled at what she saw.

"Ms. Smith, there are two beds next door that need to be made and an IV pole sitting in the hallway that needs to be put away."

I attempted to explain, but the supervisor cut me off.

"Excuse me?" The supervisor raised her eyebrows and cocked

her head as she spoke. It was clearly a sign of no reproach.

"Yes maam," looking regretfully at Mrs. Webster.

"Get going. Don't let me get you into trouble," Mrs. Webster said quietly.

I was finished making the beds before I remembered that it had been my lunch break. By that time, it wasn't.

The following day, the supervisor was as pleasant as could be when she saw me hanging out with the lunch room gang. She even joined us and we all extended the lunch break an extra ten minutes. That was acceptable. Apparently, sitting in the patient's room was not. It was then that I realized that a good nurse by this supervisor's standards was the one who was either social or visibly busy with tangible, billable and measurable services. Mrs. Moores's lonely death had made me realize that the best nursing goes beyond billable services. From then on, whenever I needed to "just talk" with my patients I made sure to keep some equipment close at hand to look busy to a casual observer. Mrs. Webster's disease progressed quickly, but this time I got my priorities straight. She did not die alone.

Mr. Davis was a middle aged gentleman in his late 50's. He had an advanced case of malignant melanoma, the deadliest form of skin cancer. The entire left side of his face and head had been eaten away by the cancerous growth, leaving necrotic, draining, foul smelling tissue where an ear, cheek and jaw had been. Despite the numerous air fresheners obtained for his room the stench would at times gag even the strongest stomachs.

Because of the smell and his constant moaning, the bed next to him was kept empty and the door to his room closed. His cancer had metastasized to his brain and liver, so there was no hope for cure or even reason to try to fix the monstrous like wound on his head.

I saw his doctor enter the room one day, and as usual, I snuck in behind him to see what I could find out. Mr. Davis made eye contact with his doctor, albeit briefly, then returned to his slow moaning.

The doctor held Mr. Davis's hand. "We'll try to get you something to be more comfortable Jim." The doctor stood silently for a moment and then left the room, tears in his eyes.

I followed him, compelled by his display of emotion. As a bedside nurse, it is easy to forget that the "order firing physicians" are also just people, many driven by this same call to make a difference, one life at a time.

"Was he a friend of yours?" I asked.

He took a deep breath. "No. He's just my patient. He was a really neat man. I never expected him to go downhill this fast. Sometimes I feel so helpless."

"Me too."

Mr. Davis didn't die quickly. I nursed him for several weeks as he continued to slowly deteriorate. One day, I needed some help turning him. Leah was the only one free.

"How can you stand it in here Karen? It reeks."

"Oh, you get used to it."

"Not me. Uggh!"

"Shhhh...", I half whispered, half gestured, "not in front of Mr. Davis. He can hear you."

"He can't hear me. Even if he can hear, he's so out of it what difference would it make? Can you finish this alone? This is disgusting."

"Yes, we'll be fine."

After Leah left, I reached down and squeezed his hand. "I'm sorry Mr. Davis."

It took a moment, but he slowly and deliberately squeezed my hand. He heard. He understood. For a brief second, I had looked through the hole in his face, right through to his soul.

Every time Henry moved, he was in excruciating pain from pancreatic cancer with metastasis to his bones. His fight against cancer was nearly complete and we all wondered why he hung on to life so feverishly, body withered, staring frightfully at the ceiling. At this point, his irregular breaths seemed more like afterthoughts. He had no visitors, so we were his only family. I was helping to change his drawsheet. I ran my fingers through his hair gently and looked deeply into his eyes.

"It's okay, Henry," I whispered in his ear. "You've fought long enough. You won't be alone."

Henry turned towards me. Our eyes met. There was a

connection that lasted for about ten seconds. Then it was gone. It faded away. He was still looking at me, still breathing, but he wasn't there. His eyes revealed only emptiness.

"That was creepy," the nurse with me said outside the room.

She had seen the distinct change too.

Henry's body died within the hour. His soul had already departed, we had seen it leave. We had felt it leave. My faith in the resurrection was reaffirmed. Being a firsthand witness made that easy.

Prioritizing a patient's psychosocial needs can be challenging, especially when you work in a unit with a lot of patients who are of sound mind but dying body. Losing several favorite patients in span of a few weeks can begin to take a toll on a nurse. Silly as it sounds, I found refuge sitting outside, communing with nature. I would sit for hours on a blanket, dog at my side, guitar in my lap like a flower child of the sixties. I began to write songs that expressed my inner flood of emotions. I called this one, "Hiding."

Hiding in between the sheets
I saw this human, so petite.
His face is pale and his hands are cold.
His mind is young but body old.

He barely moves except to breathe.
He doesn't notice when you leave.
He's always fed but he doesn't eat.
He's skin and bones, with little meat.

From needles poked his arms are blue.
As if that's all we know to do.
His eyes stay open, though he can't see.
I'm told he'll never respond to me.

For him there is no day or night,
just never ending minutes and never ending light.
Family and friends come frequently,
but tubes and body are all they see.

He lingers on, but why we ask.
It's hard to tell how long he'll last.
If only I could be the one to set him free.
To painlessness eternally.

And when the body dares to moan.
They close the doors, again alone.
They say he has no joy or pain.
They say to care is all in vain.

But here I sit and hold his hand.
And empathize as best I can.
The moaning leaves, along with life.
There's no more suffering, no more strife.

Yet, on his face is etched a smile.
I knew my efforts were worthwhile.
He lived a man and he died with pride.
For the seat was not empty by his side.

After several weeks I had produced about six songs, each progressively more depressing in both lyrics and melody. One evening when my fiancée dropped by for a visit, I proudly sang my latest composition. As I finished, I looked up, expecting the usual, "That's neat," response. Instead, his face scrunched all up and he sat back in his chair, taking a deep breath as he did so.

"Well?" I asked.

His silence betrayed his feelings.

"I thought it was good," I said defensively. "I don't care what you think. I put my guitar back in the case and closed each of the buckles with a loud snap. "Don't worry, I won't make you listen to my songs anymore."

"The song is good," he said.

"Then why the face?" I asked.

"It's just... it's just that it is so depressing. Can't you write anything... happy?"

I was taken aback by his poignant revelation. I hadn't seen my creations as the "Death Songs" that they really were. I hadn't understood how much the songs had become an outlet for my expression of grief for those patients I had lost, and for those patients I would inevitably lose as a nurse.

At the age of 22, the illusion of immortality enjoyed by my non-nursing peers had been wrenched from my grasp. I had watched people take their last breath and seen emptiness fill their staring eyes. I had washed cool, mottled skin on lifeless limp bodies. I had tied identification tags to their toes and wrapped them in plastic. I had taken them down to the morgue and put them on long metal trays, then slid them into refrigerated compartments. The sound of the refrigerator door closing, echoing on for hours in my mind, reinforced deaths' finality to me the most.

My fiancée had waited out my silence.

"I hadn't realized how much trouble I was having dealing with all this stuff at work. Have I been that depressing?"

"Well, only when you sing!"

"Thanks a heap!" I exclaimed.

The conversation changed, but more importantly, so did my attitude. I knew at that moment I would never need to write another Death Song. My repertoire was complete. Dealing with death or suffering never gets easy, but as a nurse you have no choice but to come to terms with the harsh realities that come with the territory. It is always sad, and tears are inevitable, but when you lean on God as your source of strength, each experience leaves you renewed, not drained; ready to reach out to the next patient who needs you.

Whether I was helping a patient through the dying process or just lending a listening empathetic ear, I gradually gained the confidence to practice without fear of reprisal from supervisors, fear of being unpopular with or misunderstood by some of the other nurses, or fear of potential heart ache. Sharing the psychosocial aspects of a patient's care during report would engender either a bored or uncomfortable "Anything else to report?" response or one of mirrored empathy. It was my way of feting out my comrades in caring. It was empowering to know that I was not alone. Working together, nursing with the "spirit" always made a visible difference in the lives we touched.

I found myself drawn to nursing students who coincidentally had begun to stick to me, a willing staff member, like glue. The ability to influence the open minds of these new nurses and teach them about "real" priorities was addictive. I decided to make teaching nursing a personal career goal, but with a Master's Degree the only doorway, it wouldn't be easy. Especially since I had told my college roommate to shoot me if I ever even mentioned going back to school for a Nursing Masters. From where I was then, I had a long way to go.

"What does the Lord require of you
but to act justly, and to love mercy
and to walk humbly with your God."
Micah 6:8

7

Weak Ends

Many patients in the hospital are unaware that a weekend has come. The view from the bed and the daily routine doesn't change much. But from a staff nurse's perspective, weekends, especially on the day staff, are usually short staffed nightmares.

"Sam called in," Julie told me, hanging up the phone.

"Are they sending anyone to replace him?" I asked.

"Nope. What does that leave us with?"

"You, me, 3 LPN's, and no aides," I replied.

"Glad you're in charge," she said, tossing me the clipboard. Julie had started about six months after me, giving me seniority with just over a year of experience.

"What's the census?" I asked turning to the night nurse.

"28," she said with a yawn, "but you've got four discharges this morning. We did the paperwork already."

I assigned each of nurses to patients by blocks that made sense geographically on the floor. I gave myself four patients, IV medication coverage for all the LPN's patients, in addition to the charge nurse duties, which included patient orders for all 28 patients. This would be a day roller skates would come in handy.

Leah, devoid of congeniality, was one of the LPNs on my weekend. I knew her assignment must be clearly defined from the start, as she could not be counted on for pitching in. I assigned Leah six baths and beds and also carefully spelled out her share of the additional chores; things like ice water and temperatures. Leah glanced over my shoulder.

"You've got to be kidding! You've got me running on both sides of the floor."

"Leah, I'm sorry, but we are short and this is the fairest way to do it. We all have heavy loads."

"This damn hospital is always short on the weekend. Why

don't they hire more people instead of killing us." Leah was still grumbling as she left the nurses' station to start vital signs while the rest of us heard report.

After report, I looked over my charge nurse "To Do" list. Fortunately, nothing was urgent at this point. Before I started patient care, I headed out to check the nine IV's I was responsible for. Leah was gently massaging her patient's back, when I entered to check the IV. She was talking in a very caring voice as she conversed with a frail, obviously contented old lady.

"I'll get you some fresh water for your flowers before I leave," Leah offered. "Your daughter's garden must be really beautiful."

It was just like Leah to go and do something so sweet when you were ready to dislike her.

By 9 a.m. I had finished washing and assessing three of my four patients. Mr. Wilkes was my last patient. The night nurse had said that his family members had been with him all night and that he had already had his bath at 6 a.m. He had an extremely deep wound on his bottom that required extensive dressings. I gathered the equipment I thought I would need for the dressing and hurried to Mr. Wilkes room. I was still moving quickly when I pushed against his door, but it failed to give way. The unexpected impact caused me to lose hold of my armload of supplies. They scattered in all directions including a couple of ace bandages that took off in a rolling race down the hall. Hearing the clatter outside, a gentleman opened the door and peeked out at me and my mess.

"Sorry, I was leaning against the door," he said quietly.

He quickly helped to gather the things from the floor and returned them to my arms.

"Mr. Wilkes is my father," he said in an apologetic tone. "My family is very close, as you can see."

I entered the room, slowly this time. The number of family members sequestered around their dying patriarch was too numerous to count.

"Go right ahead and do what you need to. You won't bother us," said a middle-aged woman, presumably the eldest daughter. "We've done his AM care already. I assume you are here to change the saline dressing on his sacral decubitus."

Her use of the proper terminology took me by surprise.

"Are you a nurse?" I asked.

"Ah, no," she replied.

"She thinks she is," said another.

"Let the nurse get her work done," said yet another.

Before my equipment was even out of my arms, this eldest daughter, aided by a younger girl with similar features had begun the arduous task of positioning Mr. Wilkes in anticipation of the dressing change. They exposed his buttocks to the room full of eager observers. I reached around at least four people seated in chairs in order to attempt to draw the curtain for privacy.

"Excuse me. Sorry. Sorry. Excuse me," I said.

"You don't need to close that dear, it won't bother us."

Despite their blatant breech of hospital visitation policies, I didn't necessarily want them to leave since WE were so short staffed and THEY were hands on care participants. However, I wasn't particularly excited about performing a dressing change under thirty scrutinizing eyes. I wondered how Mr. Wilkes might have felt if he had been aware that his bare bottom was being exposed to his children and grandchildren. I wasn't sure how to assert myself in a group where I was obviously outnumbered.

"Boy, you sure have a big family," was the best I could muster as an opening statement.

"The evening nurse kicked us all out, but the night nurses were great."

"We snuck back in two at a time!"

"When they found us, they told us we could stay as long as we were quiet."

I still hadn't opened any of my dressings. I leaned over and covered Mr. Wilkes buttocks.

"How's he doing?" I asked.

"The doctor doesn't expect him to last the week."

I excused myself back over and around the bed in order to see his face. I held his hand.

"Mr. Wilkes, I'm Karen, your nurse today. You are lucky to have such a wonderful loving family around you."

I listened to his heart and lungs. Not that it did anything, but it seemed to comfort the family to know their dad was being tended to.

"Sounds okay," I told them.

"Mr. Wilkes, I need to change your dressing on your bottom."

After a final hand squeeze, I side stepped and excused myself back to the dressing change position.

"Can you reach the curtain for me?" I asked the woman behind me.

"Why don't we all get a cup of coffee and let this gal get her work done?" the son guarding the door suggested.

As if on cue, all the others stood and exited the room, single file, each thanking me as they left. Only the eldest daughter remained to help.

"What's that white shiny thing there?" the daughter asked, pointing inside the deep wound.

"Bone," I replied.

"Oh," she said matter of factly.

"Are you doing okay?" I asked.

"I'm fine. I help any of the girls that will let me. It makes me feel like I'm doing something. It's so hard to just sit and watch him."

"This must be very difficult for you."

"It's been a long year." She shared how he had cared for their mom for years explaining why they wouldn't leave him now. As I left the room, the entire Wilkes family was walking back down the hall, en masse, coffee in hand.

Leah, the LPN stopped them and said, "I'm sorry, visiting hours aren't until noon. Besides that, only four visitors are allowed at a time. The rest will have to wait downstairs."

I joined Leah and said quietly to her, "It's okay, Leah. Special exception. They aren't in our way."

I motioned for them to pass.

"Thanks," they said and quietly returned to the room.

After they had all passed, Leah turned to me and said, "You better hope the supervisor doesn't see this."

"I do believe that the visitation policy allows for exceptions at the nurse's discretion."

"How can you stand it?" Leah asked. "I hate it when those big families move in. The rooms are small enough without them. I always kick them out."

"They weren't so bad. Actually, the daughter helped me with Mr. Wilkes dressing."

"I wouldn't do that. Next thing you know they'll sue the hospital saying that we were so inadequately staffed they had to provide care."

"We are inadequately staffed," I countered.

"It's your license boss," she said sarcastically. "I'm just telling you what I've seen. They are wonderful to your face and then they stab you in the back," Leah said voicing her bitterness on the subject as she left, insuring that she would get the last word in.

I entered the station to find that a mountain of charts had gathered on the desk in my absence. Most of them had physician orders that required prompt attention and processing. It was difficult and time consuming without a secretary on the weekends to help. Inevitably, the most important orders were hidden at the bottom of the pile.

One of Mr. Wilkes kids walked past the station, which reminded me to find the family visitation regulations in the hospital policy book. There were several overstuffed three-ring binders to sieve through. I had just found the policy in Section III B.2.e. in the second binder when Leah came into the station. The book was too heavy to move quickly out of her eagerly inquiring eyes.

"Bet I'm right," she said.

I ignored her and kept reading, looking for any phrase to support my decision. The limits to four visitors within certain time limits were clearly stated.

"Ah ha! Blah, blah, blah... it says, at the discretion of the nurse in charge. I thought so. Here you read it."

"I don't need to read the damn policy. That's your job. You're in charge. If you want twenty family members hanging around all day, who am I to stop you? I'm going to lunch."

As she walked away and down the hall, I could hear her continue the conversation with herself, "even if you're nuts and you'll probably get sued. It's not my license. If it were me, I'd boot every last one of them out of here."

I grabbed a piece of uneaten apple pie from a patient's tray and ate it in the nurses' station. Julie entered, looking harried.

"Lunch," I said with my mouth half full. "I saw another piece on 2O B's if you want some.

"Is it good?"

"It's food."

"Nevermind. I have a sandwich."

"Go get it and sit a minute."

"Alright."

Julie returned momentarily and sat next to me. She ate quietly, staring at her sandwich.

"What's up? You seem a little upset."

"I'm too embarrassed to even talk about it."

"Julie, what's up?"

"You know Zach in 12 B?"

"Boy do I know Zach!"

Zach was a 22 year old recovering from a severe car accident. He had fractured both legs, which were being treated with pins and traction. He also had multiple facial fractures, including his jaw, which was wired shut. He had been on a respirator for several weeks, but was breathing fine on his own now and was on the road to recovery. Zach spent his idle time reading pornographic magazines supplied by his buddies and flirting with the nurses.

"What did Zach say to you?" I asked.

"He said it was the nurses' job to make him, you know…," Julie hesitated a moment before she finished, "take care of him, you know..." She paused again. "I don't really have to do that do I?"

Zach had spotted a naive nurse and had gone for broke.

"I'm gonna kill him," was my response, standing as I spoke.

"Wait, wait," she said grabbing my arm and pulling me back to my chair. "I think you better cool down first. He's going to be embarrassed enough as it is. I'm just relieved I don't really have to do that."

"Ughgh!" we chimed simultaneously.

"I've been taking care of him since he came from the ICU," I shared. "At first he kept exposing himself a little to me, pretending like it was an accident. I caught on to his tricks quickly and tossed a towel to cover him. That stopped it. Then he tried to get me to wash his privates when I helped him with his bath."

"What did you do?"

"I handed him the washcloth and reminded him that though

his jaw and leg were broken, his arm wasn't."

"He did it?"

"No problem."

Julie stood up. "I'm going to kill him for you."

"Yo, yo, yo!" I held Julie's arm and sat her down.

"He told me the nurses always did it since his ribs were bruised and it hurt to bend."

"You know, if he was fifty years older we'd laugh and say what a dirty old man he is. But having him so close to our own ages makes it different somehow."

"More uncomfortable."

"Gross."

"Definitely gross," Julie concurred.

The sexualization of nurses in our society creates a complex nuance when it comes to the provision of cross-gender intimate personal care. Nurses unfortunately have to deal with men (or women) patients who test the boundaries of propriety on a regular basis.

"Do I seemed cooled down enough to have a constructive conversation with our dirty young man Zach?"

"Not yet," she said half laughing, half furious. "I'm so angry!"

"He had a lot of nerve. Next time Julie, trust your instincts! You know better."

"Well after we had to put real leeches on that guys leg last week, I wasn't sure what to believe."

"That was really disgusting."

"Even more for me," she replied. "I had to do it."

"You made out alright in that trade," I said grinning. "You drive a hard bargain as I recall."

I had traded Julie four patients for the one with the leeches.

"I didn't want to do it either," she reminded me.

"I'm going to talk with Zach. Ready or not, here I come!"

As the door opened, I could see Zach grinning as usual, reading one of his magazines. He took one look at me and his face immediately changed expression, like a kid with a hand caught in the cookie jar. I slowly closed the door behind me.

"We need to talk," I began.

He didn't say a word. I walked over and stood at the side of his bed.

"Zach you were out of line with Julie."

"I know. Well, nothing ventured, nothing gained," Zach said smugly breaking the silence, through his wired jaw, enunciating every word with his lips.

"She's a very nice girl and you've made her very upset."

"I'm sorry."

I dragged the chair from the corner of the room up close to his bed and sat down.

"What were you thinking? You must have known you wouldn't get away with it."

I stayed silent. Seconds of eternity seemed to pass.

"Do you realize how long I've been in this place?"

"I know it's been a while."

"Six weeks in ICU, three of which I can't remember. Tomorrow will mark my third week here. I had a great sex life before this accident. Basically, I'm just horny."

"I'm sure reading porn magazines all day isn't helping matters much."

"Maybe not." He paused to gather his thoughts. "You know, you lay here week after week eating ground up spaghetti and meatballs through a straw and you wonder. Will I ever be normal? Will my jaw work? Will my leg heal? Will I be able to have sex?"

"Nothing vital to your sexual functioning was injured. There's no reason why your sex life will be impaired."

"Well, I've tried a couple of times to, you know, to see if it would still work. But it doesn't. That never happened to me before, ever. Believe me."

I was taken aback. This was a component of Zach's needs I hadn't considered in my nursing care plan. He was "living" this hellish experience, I had just been "observing" from my own "intact" life. Regardless of his earlier behavior, he deserved our empathy.

"Perhaps knowing that a nurse or visitor could burst into the room at any time might have had something to do with that?"

"I hope you're right."

"Maybe there is something we can do to help." I checked my watch. "Are you expecting visitors this afternoon?"

"Nope. What are you proposing?"

"I'm here until 3:3O. What if I could guarantee you absolutely no interruptions for an hour this afternoon."

"You mean it?"

"On one condition."

"Yeah?"

"No more harassing my nurses. Do we have a deal?"

"Yup!" His grin had returned. "Can I call my girlfriend?"

"That's your business," I said standing to leave. I walked to his bedside stand. "How about switching back to these motorcycle magazines for awhile too?"

"You said only one condition."

"Zach...?" I said, drawing out the last syllable.

"Okay."

"And you owe Julie an apology."

"That's three."

"So it is." I was grinning this time. "Call me when you're ready for the blockade."

"Okay."

I was barely out the door when I heard Zach call me back.

"What Zach?"

"Thanks."

I winked in response. Julie met me in the hall outside the room. I beckoned for her to join me somewhere more private. I shared what happened.

"Do you have time to make a sign for the door?"

"What would it say?"

"Well, we certainly won't put what's actually going on in there!"

"How about: "Treatment in Progress"?"

"That won't keep staff out."

We settled for "Do not open door 2-3 p.m. Absolutely no visitors or staff allowed."

"Are you done with your assignment yet?" I asked.

She gave me an update. Her noon meds were already 2O minutes late and she still had beds to make. Leah walked past. I turned to her.

"Leah, would you mind helping out Julie a little. The beds in 18 need to be changed."

She stopped and scowled.

"Yes, I would mind. I've got my own assignment, which is quite sufficient, and I'm in the middle of Mrs. Gray's bath. When I'm done with that, I'm going for a cigarette. Maybe I'll have time later, and then again, maybe I won't. I'm not going to promise anything." Leah left, before counter-discussion could begin.

I rolled my eyes. Julie laughed and shook her head.

"Julie, go get your meds done. I have a minute. Are the sheets in there?"

"Yes. Are you sure you have time?"

"No problem."

The beds only took me a few minutes then I headed out on IV rounds. I was especially concerned about one of my IV's that had been running irregularly all day. Entering the room this time, I understood why. Leah was standing at the IV bag, adjusting the drops.

"Looks a little slow," she said casually.

"Leah, can I speak to you in the hall a second?" I kept my voice nonchalant so as not to alarm the patient. She joined me in the hall. "Leah, you're not supposed to be adjusting the IV's. That is outside your scope of practice."

"None of the other girls mind when I keep their IV's on time."

"I mind. This IV has been running erratically all day."

"This is the first time I touched it. You can't blame me for that."

I didn't believe her, but having no other proof, I knew better than to confront her further at this time.

"If that's the way you want it, fine. See if I care if your IV's run dry."

"Leah," I said, side-stepping, "I certainly would appreciate it if you would let me know of any IV's that don't look right to your experienced eye."

"Watching the IV's is your job, not mine. I'm not getting paid to do that."

"I'm not asking you to watch my IV's," I said getting frustrated.

"Of course not. You don't even trust me to do what I've been doing longer than you've been a nurse."

In the field of medicine, titles rule, and experience is welcomed but not honored. The pecking order is very clearly and legally delineated.

"It's not that I don't think you are capable, it's just that since I'm ultimately responsible for the IV, I would prefer to do the adjusting."

"Yeah right." Leah walked away.

"I'm sorry," I called after her.

I had become apologetic around Leah, not a sign of self-confidence in a leader. While she was without doubt in the wrong on this particular policy, I was oblivious to how selective I had been with stretching the boundaries of policy adherence this busy weekend day with supervisors few and far between. I was too green of a manager to recognize how important it was to make hard working employees like Leah feel appreciated. A different approach might have made her my ally, not more cantankerous. I lacked the experience to recognize how crucial every set of eyes and hands are in short staffed situations. I could have just taught her how to check the IV properly.

As I returned to the nurses' station, I spotted Zach's girlfriend. She was dressed in a cute little outfit and was grinning sheepishly as she entered Zach's room. Checking my watch, I saw it was 1:45. Julie emerged from the medication room.

"Finish the sign yet?" I asked.

"Just now, it's in the med room."

"His girlfriend is here."

"I'll go hang the sign."

I was finishing my charting when Leah came around the corner.

"Why can't anyone go in Zach's room until 3:3O?" Leah asked innocently.

"He doesn't want to be disturbed. He hasn't had a good rest in awhile."

Leah looked at me quizzically. I went back to my charting. Unfortunately, Zach's girlfriend snuck out of the room a few minutes later. Leah wiggled her eyebrows and smirked.

"Wo, wo, wo! I know what they're gonna do!" she said.

"Just keep it quiet Leah," I whispered.

Fortunately, she didn't ask me about the policy for this.

The phone rang with the news of two admissions that would arrive before the change of shift, one a transfer from the ER. As I hung up the phone, I turned to see several nurses in ER scrubs standing next to a patient on a stretcher. One nurse was readjusting the IV rate. The other nurse was making a brief note on her stack of papers. The man was obese and had a stomach tube protruding from his nose.

"Who wants report?" asked the gal with the clipboard.

"What room?" the other called.

"You are not getting me to do an admission this late, so don't even ask," Leah whispered in my ear.

"What room?" the nurse asked again impatiently as I checked the census report. "I don't have all day."

"Oh..uhh..let's put him in 16A," I said after a pause. "Sorry, I just found out you were coming a minute ago."

"He's been in the ER since early this morning and real anxious to get up here."

I peeked at the chart to see his name.

"Hi Mr. Cajun. I'm Karen, welcome to the 5th floor."

"It's about god damn time. How soon before the TV can be hooked up?"

"We'll do our best," I said as the ER nurses and I rolled him down the hall.

"Watch it, watch it," he clamored when the stretcher graced the door frame as we swung into his room.

When we loosened the cover sheet in preparation to transfer Mr. Cajun to his bed, the source for some of his bitterness quickly became apparent. Mr. Cajun was an above the knee bilateral amputee. It was obvious from the multitude of scar lines on both leg stumps, that he was nostranger to the hospital environment.

"You people forget we are here."

The ER nurse replied, "Nobody could miss you, Mr. Cajun.

"Wait!" he called as we prepared to transfer him using a pull sheet underneath of him. "Doesn't anyone even stop to talk to the patient? I'm not a bundle of wood you know. I'm in a lot of pain, which you would know if you ever bothered to read the chart."

"Mr. Cajun, your chart just arrived with you," I said in defense.

"I've been here in the hospital for five hours already and I'll bet you don't even know why I'm here, and yet you're ready to jump in and move me."

Touché' I thought, then asked, "Mr. Cajun, what should I know before I move you?"

"If you can be patient a minute, an impossibility for most health care workers," he said in a sarcastic tone, "I'll move off the stretcher by myself. Get the bed a little lower...and make sure the tube in my nose can reach. These things are really tender!" He continued with a series of directions until he was safely in the new bed. "Now you all can leave and don't come back till you've read my chart and know why I'm here AND when my TV will be hooked up."

I got a brief report from the ER nurses back in the station, then wearing big smiles they booked. "He is all yours. Good riddance!"

It was clear that they had run up to the floor with him the minute that he'd been assigned to a floor by the admitting office. From a nurse's perspective, there is a fine line between assertiveness and annoyance. Nurses aren't always up to the challenges of a demanding patient, especially at the end of a busy weekend day.

Mr. Cajun was a diabetic with Crohn's disease, a chronic recurring inflammatory disease of the bowel. According to his history, he had spent about half of the last five years in the hospital. He was being admitted for a bowel obstruction, his third time this year. He had lost his legs over ten years ago in a motorcycle accident. He lived alone in an apartment, and held down a full-time job with a trucking firm. After double checking his orders, phoning the TV lady and gathering the equipment to attach his nose tube to wall suction, I dragged the blood pressure machine with my foot down the hall and ventured back into 16A. He was busy unpacking his toiletries into his overbed tray storage. He looked up as I entered.

"I was wondering if I was going to have to hook myself up to suction."

"No, that's why they pay me the big bucks," I replied.

"I'm sure you're just raking it in here," he said in belittling tone.

I installed the wall suction apparatus, checked to make sure his tube was properly placed, and then attached the suction tubing to his nose tubing.

"Bet you don't know why I have this tube," Mr. Cajun baited me.

"Because you have an obstruction."

"Lucky guess."

"No," I replied confidently. "This is your third obstruction this year because of your Crohns.

Mr. Cajun looked surprised.

"I read your chart, Mr. Cajun. Is there anything else you want to ask me?"

He raised his middle finger at me in retort.

"Nice," I replied.

In the real world outside the hospital, nasty gestures or remarks would automatically generate an equivocal response. But in the surreal hospital environment, nurses learn to curtail natural impulses and to look past patient unpleasantness.

"Are you in any pain Mr. Cajun?"

"Not now. Only when those idiot doctors took turns pressing on my abdomen."

"They are only doing their job."

"Sure, maybe the first guy. But the next five residents didn't have to push so damn hard. Either they really don't have a clue to how uncomfortable it is for a patient or they don't give a damn."

"It must be frustrating for you. I can see from your chart that you don't need a lot of orientation to our hospital routine."

"No, I don't think so. You are new around here; I don't recognize you from my last admission."

"I've been here a year."

"Do you know what you're doing?"

"They've got me in charge," I responded confidently.

"That's a real comfort," he sneered. "Did you take care of the TV?"

"I wouldn't have come back in here if I hadn't."

"Alright, maybe you've got a chance."

After I finished checking his vital signs and verifying the IV, I began to leave.

"I know it's close to the change of shift and I won't see a soul for another hour unless I fall asleep, so before you go would you..." Mr. Cajun proceeded to provide me with a 15 minute laundry list of things to do before I escaped back to the main desk.

The evening crew was already filing in.

"Karen, the other admission came while you were in with Mr. Cajun," the oncoming nurse shared. "I'll go check her out."

"Music to my ears. Yes, I'd really appreciate it," glancing at Leah while I spoke.

Julie asked, "Did you get the admission sheet done on Mr. Cajun?"

"He's set up and I've got his vital signs, but I didn't finish all the paperwork."

"I'm almost done charting. I'll finish it while you get report going."

"Thanks, I'd appreciate that Julie. But before you go in, let me give you his history quick or he'll put you through the ringer."

"Nothing will faze me after the day I've had," she replied.

After report was done I finished my charting and made a belated final round before officially signing off.

"Oh I thought you were long gone," one patient remarked checking her watch. Aren't you off at three?"

"Only in the movies."

The evening nurses were in the process of kicking out the Wilkes family, in keeping with the hospital policy. My pleas during report had obviously fallen on deaf ears. Several family members thanked me on their way past. The eldest daughter stopped and asked me if I was on tomorrow.

"Yes. I'm sorry that you aren't being allowed to stay."

"Don't worry, we'll be back," she winked devilishly.

Julie emerged from Mr. Cajun's room.

"I thought you, were out of here," I remarked. "Did he give you a hard time?"

"At first, but after the day I've had, I just held to my task and ignored his comments."

"Good for you."

"Are we having fun yet?"

"Nothing they teach you in school can prepare you for days like this."

"If they did, everyone would quit!"

"Let's get out of here."

We grabbed our coats and gear from the station and arm in arm pulled each other up the hallway. Spotting Zach's now open door we simultaneously came to an abrupt halt and retreated. We poked our heads in the door. Seeing both of us, Zach began to laugh. He then grinned widely and indicated two thumbs up.

"Good night Zach!" I called.

"See you in the morning Zach," Julie chimed in.

"We are out of here!" emphasizing each word.

I checked my watch. 4:15. At least with the weekend day shift you could look forward to a Saturday evening social life, that is until 8 or 9 when your body faded from exhaustion! The alarm would sound early. Sunday's shift, only 13 hours away, could only promise more of the same.

"Let us not become weary in doing good,
for at the proper time we will reap a harvest if we do
not give up. Therefore, as we have opportunity,
let us do good to all people."

Galatians 6:9-10

8

Dr. Goliath Meets Nurse Davey

"What did you say?" asked Mr. Appleby, a 53 year old man with a recently diagnosed brain tumor.

This was the first time I had noticed he had difficulty hearing me. Hearing loss is a possible side effect of certain tumors depending on their location in the brain. But Mr. Appleby had a cerebella tumor, affecting his coordination and movement, which made this finding unlikely. I asked his wife if he had any history of hearing problems, which she denied.

"I noticed it today too," she said.

"I'll mention it to Dr. Benjamin when he comes in later," I told her.

Dr. Benjamin was a big, burly non-approachable type of guy. He was in his late sixties and clearly remembered the days when nurses stood up whenever physicians entered the station and never questioned a physician's judgment. So it didn't surprise me when he told me Mr. Appleby's hearing seemed fine to him.

Several days later, the hearing loss became even more pronounced. I began to wonder if the hearing loss could have something to do with one of his medications. He had been receiving injections of Gentamycin for several weeks to treat a stubborn infection. Remembering details about medications wasn't easy. I was forever looking up the same drugs over and over again. But the association of Gentamycin and hearing loss was one drilled into me from school, so I ventured back to Dr. Benjamin to check if this was something we might want to explore.

"Doctor, I was asking because I noticed Mr. Appleby has been on the Gentamycin way beyond the time recommended in the PDR." PDR is the nickname for Physician's Desk Reference, the most commonly used medication reference.

Dr. Benjamin pushed away from the desk and stood to his full height of over six feet. "I don't know where you nurses get off thinking you can tell a doctor who's gone through 12 years of training, what drug YOU think MY patient should or shouldn't get. When you get your medical degree then you can offer ME your advice. Until then, mind your own business!" With that, he stormed out of the station.

My head nurse, Mrs. Staples, had overheard part of the conversation and joined me after he left. "What's he all upset about?"

"I questioned him about one of his patients."

"You're brave to try that with Dr. Benjamin. Which patient?"

"I'm really concerned about Mr. Appleby's hearing loss. I think it may have something to do with the fact that he's been on Gentamycin so long."

"Let me see." We walked to the cart where the medication records were kept. Looking at Mr. Appleby's record we saw that he had been receiving the injections three times a day for over six weeks now.

"Did Dr. Benjamin think it was okay?" she asked.

"Yes, but I don't think that Dr. Benjamin would stop the injections now even if he did agree with me. He's not the kind of doctor that can handle a nurse looking over his shoulder."

"Well, you've told him. It's his patient. I wouldn't worry about it. It's probably fine."

"But Mrs. Staples, Mr. Appleby is going deaf! Am I supposed to ignore that?"

"The man has a brain tumor Karen. There is no way to know for sure that isn't the cause of the deafness."

The phone rang, ending the conversation. I had the weekend off, so I let it drop.

The next time I saw Mr. Appleby, I was working evening shift. His wife was sitting beside him when I entered the room.

"How's Mr. Appleby doing tonight?"

"He's so frustrated about not being able to hear very well. I asked Dr. Benjamin about it and he said it was the tumor. He was doing so well until this. It's really quite a setback."

"I'm sure it's tough on all of you."

I knew better than to mention my concerns about the medicine to her. If she said anything to Dr. Benjamin, he would know it came from me. The last thing Mrs. Appleby needed was to lose faith in the physician whom at this point was her only source of hope.

When I checked his medications, sure enough, the Gentamycin was still being given, around the clock. I was scheduled to give the next dose at 8 p.m. As I prepared the medication around 7:30, I knew that I would not be able to administer the drug to him in good conscious. So now what? I called Dr. Benjamin.

"Dr. Benjamin, this is Karen on 5. I need to inform you that I will not be giving Mr. Appleby's Gentamycin injection this evening."

"Why not?"

Taking a deep breath I went on. "Mr. Appleby is continuing to shows signs of ototoxicity, which is a common side effect of the Gentamycin, so I am going to hold it."

The voice on the other end of the phone exploded. "The hell you are. We've had this conversation already. I'm his doctor. You are the nurse. I'm ordering the medication to be continued."

"Doctor, I'm the only nurse on duty this evening and I'm informing you that I do not intend to give him the drug for reasons already stated. If you want him to have it you are welcome to come and give it yourself."

"You are not the only nurse in the hospital capable of giving an injection. I suggest you find someone." With that he hung up the phone.

I called the supervisor on duty and she told me she would be up shortly. When she arrived, I recapped the situation for her. Like Mrs. Staples had done, the supervisor reviewed the chart and PDR information.

"What's the big deal? He's had so many injections already. The doctor is well aware of the information you've presented and feels the medication is warranted."

"I'm sorry to cause problems, but I cannot in good conscious give this medication. The PDR guidelines are clear. It has to stop somewhere."

The supervisor sighed deeply and shook her head. She started towards the medication cart.

"What are you going to do?" I asked.

"I'm going to give it."

"That's too bad," I said.

"I don't have any choice. Who else is going to give it?"

"I was hoping that no one would."

I didn't tell Mrs. Appleby what was going on at that point. First of all, I had no idea if I was going to get anywhere; secondly, I wasn't sure now if I was right about the hearing loss. Having no support from people who had more experience than me made me question my own conclusions. When I passed report to nights, they raised their eyebrows. Having seen me start the ball rolling on this issue, and agreeing with my observations, they weren't sure what they would do with the nighttime dose.

The next evening, the floor was buzzing with gossip of how I had taken on Dr. Benjamin. Nights had joined forces with me, making their supervisor come and give the 4 a.m. injection. The supervisors were angry with us for making waves. Dr. Benjamin had called in to the Director of Nurses to complain. I was told to expect a visit from the top supervisor. I didn't have to wait long.

"Karen, I'd like to have a word with you." The Director was white haired with glasses hanging from a silver chain that nestled in between her buxom chest. Her uniform was heavily starched and noticeably devoid of the wear and tear generally seen on those nurses in the trenches.

"Dr. Benjamin is extremely upset over yesterday's incident. He feels that his judgment is being inappropriately questioned. Dr. Benjamin has a wonderful reputation and has been at Main Hospital for many years. We would like to ask you to honor his requests."

"I'm sorry I've caused so much trouble, but as I've told the others, I cannot follow this particular order in good faith. I have no difficulty with anything else Dr. Benjamin has asked."

"Karen, you have to do it."

"No, I don't believe that I do. I'm giving you adequate warning that I will hold the medicine again this evening."

The elderly woman's jugular vein became more pronounced as she continued. "I don't see why you are going to make the busy evening supervisor come up just to give a routine injection. The patient's going to get it anyway, whether you give it or not. You could save everyone a lot of bother if you just gave it."

"I realized how wrong it was to give yesterday. It's no different today. You do what you have to. I'll do what I have to."

The supervisor left me and had a brief discussion with Mrs. Staples before leaving the unit, noticeably smiling at everyone but me. Mrs. Staples sweetly attempted to convince me to change my mind, but her passive personality was no match for my determination. Secretly I think she admired my courage.

The evening supervisor dutifully came at 8:OO to administer the medication, as did the supervisor for the night shift's dose. By the next day, the day shift had begun to get nervous about giving the now highly questioned medication and made the boycott universal. Even some of the supervisors admitted their level of discomfort with the continued use of the medicine, but they felt their hands were tied. Dr. Benjamin was a powerful man at the hospital.

The next evening when my supervisor came to give the medicine, she paused at the medication cart, then wrote "HOLD" where the nurse is supposed to initial that the dose was given.

"I'm really tired of coming up here," she said to me. "I've got more important things to do."

She glared at me, then left the unit.

Finally! It had taken three days, but I had worn them down. The supervisors got the chief of medical staff involved who spoke to Dr. Benjamin and asked him to put an end to this unnecessary waste of staff time. The medicine was promptly discontinued.

It took several more days, but Mr. Appleby did gradually regain his hearing. Mr. Appleby told me, "It was driving me nuts not hearing what was going on!"

Mrs. Appleby joined in, "It was so strange, I wonder why his hearing came and went like that? Do you think it will happen again?"

"I doubt it Mrs. Appleby. He should be better now."

Once I returned to the day shift, the unavoidable reunion was inevitable. Dr. Benjamin was sitting in the station when I sped around the corner, as usual, going too fast to change direction. I nonchalantly took at seat at the desk and started charting. He looked up at me, then back down into his chart. He would talk to me when he was good and ready. The other staff members would enter the station, see the two of us, raise their eyebrows and evacuate before the storm hit. Eventually, Dr. Benjamin rose to leave, but paused next to my chair.

"Well, you got what you wanted. Are you happy?" He spoke in a sarcastic tone.

"Yes I am as a matter of fact. Have you seen Mr. Appleby? He's doing great now that his hearing is coming back."

"There was nothing to come back. I told you, he didn't have a hearing problem to start with." He walked out of the station feeling like a winner.

I sat there, smiling. As soon as he had turned the corner and entered the elevator, the staff returned cheering. I felt like a winner.

But the real winner had been Mr. Appleby.

"If a ruler's anger rises against you,
do not leave your post,
calmness can lay great errors to rest."

Ecclesiastes 10:4

9

Basic Lessons

Nursing is a career that provides you with daily opportunities to look stupid. But using the glass half full philosophy of life, it also means that you learn something new every day.

After 18 months working on the medical surgical unit, I transferred to the hospitals ICU ward in search of an excitement fix. Without even reading the sign, you could tell that you were entering a critical care unit as you exited the elevator and began to walk the narrow hallway that led to the unit. The sea green walls were tiled, adding a chill not present on the regular floors. The absence of windows created an eerie glow of dim light. The air was still. The sounds of high pitched machine alarms and chimes occasionally spliced through the constant beat of heart monitors in dueling syncopation.

Staff members bustled around, quietly and seriously attending to their patients. Physicians read their charts with intense focus. The nurse manager exuded competence and confidence. Gaiety came in quiet bursts, not noticeable to the casual observer. This was professional nursing at a technical peak.

Ten patient rooms circled a glass walled nurses' station. Pictures were replaced by monitors and oxygen hookups. Some rooms were so filled with equipment that they were standing room only. Gravely ill patients laid propped in the beds with so many IV and monitor lines attached to them that they looked like marionettes.

Walking into the ICU ward one evening, I spotted a patient wearing high top sneakers and a football helmet. I couldn't wait to hear report on this wacko. The hospital was small enough to have only one critical unit, so we saw everything, including an occasional psychologically disturbed client.

"Mrs. Dearborne, 51, admitted for a gastrointestinal bleed secondary to an esophogeal tear, patient of A, M and R's, has a Blakemore (stomach) tube in place. 3OO cc of coffee ground material in the suction at O6OO. Irrigate the tube with normal saline q 4. IV's at... Here's her medication sheet. Vital signs are stable. That's about it."

"Come on. What about her psychiatric status?" I asked, thinking they had forgotten the juicy part.

"I don't know anything. She seemed fine to me." Deb looked serious.

"Yeah, right. You're pulling my leg."

"Honest, I have no idea what you are talking about." Deb looked over to her counterpart, "Hey, does Mrs. Dearborne have a psychiatric history? You had her yesterday didn't you?"

The nurse looked up from her charting. "Psych history? That's news to me too. The doctor was looking into alcohol abuse because of the diagnosis, but both she and her family swear she doesn't drink! She's really a nice lady. Why do you ask?"

"Karen, thought she had a psych history."

"You two must be in cahoots!" I said, shaking my head.

Surely there was a story behind the helmet and the sneakers. These two had a reputation as big kidders. I looked at the both of them, but they only returned blank stares. They were good. I dropped it, deciding to wait for them to crack.

"Okay Deb, what about this next guy?"

It was fairly straight forward stuff for ICU. He was a patient with end-stage pulmonary disease on a respirator. The big machines with all the dials, gauges and alarms had overwhelmed me at first. I was afraid that I would trip over the electric cord, or inadvertently disconnect the tubing at one of the many junctions, or not be able to put on sterile gloves fast enough to suction a patient before they smothered. One day I did accidentally trip and pull out the plug, only to discover the machine had an automatic battery reserve. Once I realized that the built-in early warning alarm systems made it difficult to harm the patient, I finally began to relax.

"What are his secretions like?" I asked.

Nurses are interested in four main things, sputum, feces, puke and blood. It is partly clinical and partly protective. We want to know what we need to brace ourselves for mentally, physically, and nasally! To survive in nursing, you must be able to tolerate at least three out of the main four without noticeable facial grimacing.

My third critical patient was an unstable post-op. Three critical care patients were tough to manage even when they were in the same room. As ICU nurse in my ward, you did baths, beds, vital signs, treatments, and medication preparation and administration. In addition to care, we were in charge of our own patients. This meant dealing with doctors and coordinating patient services with other departments, from the lab to social services. Depending on the severity of each critical patient, a nurse might only be able to safely care for one or two.

Report ended without hint of Mrs. Dearborne or her problem.

"Is that everything?" I asked.

"That's all. Doesn't look too bad."

I gathered my papers, figuring they would stop me in the doorway to let me in on the "gag". When I was almost out the door, an inexperienced aide on my shift, Trixie, entered the report room.

"What's the helmet doing on the patient in Room 2?" Trixie asked innocently.

Debbie explained, "She has a stomach tube tied to it. The doctor is using the helmet to help put some traction on the tube to hold it in position within her stomach. It's a great idea. It is much more comfortable than when use tape on the nose for traction."

"She looks really silly wearing the sneakers and the helmet," Trixie added.

"The high top sneaks keep her from getting foot-drop contractures. Mrs. Dearborne spends a lot of time in bed because of emphysema. She brought them in from home."

Debbie continued on with her charting. I left quickly, hoping that they wouldn't piece together my ignorance. I learned something new, and as always, I learned it the hard way.

The evening progressed routinely until shortly before 1O p.m. when the sounds of rolling thunder and distant booms began to pierce the inner confines of our windowless unit. The lights flickered momentarily in sequence with the loudest bangs, simultaneously setting off a round of alarms on monitoring equipment. Alone in my room of three patients, I sought the advice of a more experienced nurse across the hall.

"Question one. Can we lose power?" I asked her.

"Yes," Nancy replied matter-of-factly. She had two patients on respirators, one of whom she was suctioning.

"Question two. What happens then? Is there back-up?"

"That's two questions."

A louder and closer bang vibrated the building, again with a flickering of lights.

"That was close. We'll have lights, but not enough power to run the equipment. Keep your patients calm. The generator will kick on after a few minutes."

"What about the respirators?"

"Get ready to bag your respirator patient."

"You've got two. What are you going to do?"

"I already called Respiratory Therapy. Speaking of the devil." Nancy nodded at Rich as he entered the room.

"Call me a devil and see if I help you bag your patient," Rich responded.

"Sorry to wake you," Nancy teased.

"You have a lot of nerve to disturb my beauty sleep."

"You'll need a lot more than sleep to attain beauty status!"

The two sounded more like feuding siblings than co-workers, perhaps justified by the tension of the moment. I returned to my room as if to prepare for battle. I gathered the football size ambu bag, hooked it to oxygen tubing, and waited at my patient's side, holding his hand for our mutual reassurance.

As the storm raged on, I began to feel a little over-reactive. I left the equipment in place and ventured over to do some routine monitoring of my other patients. I was in the middle of emptying a urinary drainage bag when the final boom struck. The lights flickered on, off, on, off, on, then off. The droning machines whirred to a stop. For a unit, usually filled with an incredible amount of white noise, the silence was overpowering and frightening. As the dim emergency lights eerily illuminated the room, I reassured the patients that everything would be okay.

"The hospital has a back-up generator that will come on in a few minutes. Please don't worry."

I returned to my patient's side, thankful that my equipment was ready to go and began the manual inflation of his lungs. 1, 2, 3, 4, Breathe, Repeat ...

A few minutes later the lights tried to come back on creating a temporary flurry of machine start up noise and alarms, then again silence. Silence except for the sounds of the nurses calling back and forth between rooms.

"Are you okay in there, Karen?"

"In control. Nancy are you and Rich behaving?"

"I am but she's not," Rich responded.

Mrs. Dearborne, the lady with the helmet and sneakers, was great. She began to tell funny stories that helped all of us stay calm. Finally after about twenty minutes, the power surged on and I was able to return my patient to the security of his respirator. I finished my end of shift chores and was preparing to pass report when the Code Alarm sounded.

"Room 7!"

The team of nurses bounced into action, one more time.

"Why do the patient's always wait until change of shift to code?" Nancy remarked, passing me with the code cart at the maximum speed limit.

I grabbed the defibrillator cart and joined in pursuit. Tammy, the nurse assigned to the patient, had already placed a board under the upper torso of the elderly man and was at the end of her first set of heart compressions when we entered.

"What's the story Tammy?"

"Post-op colon resection. Going downhill all night. Lungs filled up with fluid. History of COPD. Went V-Fib on me."

Simply translated, her patient had a cardiac arrest triggered by respiratory failure.

I set up the defibrillator, lubricated the pads and stood ready near the chest. In the meantime, another RN had taken over respirations, and Tammy promptly switched her compression rate to a two-man CPR rate. The nurse expertly timed her breaths to coincide with Tammy's pauses in chest compressions as though it had been choreographed. A sleepy resident who had been jettisoned back into full wakefulness by the ringing code alarm throughout the unit, grabbed the endotracheal airway tube Nancy had pulled from the code cart drawer as he walked past her. He looked at the monitor as he moved to the head of the bed.

"4OO watts?"

"Ready," I quickly replied.

"Go."

Tammy stopped compressions, I positioned the pads on the man's chest.

"Stand clear," I warned.

Everyone checked their position and stood back from the bed. I pressed the buttons on the defibrillator and watched the patient's body jolt downward then upward from the charge. All eyes watched the cardiac monitor. The line went from wavy back to straight.

"Again," the resident ordered.

"Charging, charging," I said watching my defibrillator gauge. "Ready. Stand clear."

Again the body jolted several inches off the bed.

"We have a rhythm," the resident called, "give him an amp of Epi."

The resident took the headboard off the bed and as if by instinct alone, inserted the tube with ease through the mouth into the patient's windpipe. Rich rounded the bend with a new respirator, parked it at the door, then squished past the rest of us in time to hook up the oxygen to the ambu bag he had brought stuffed under his arm.

"It's in," the resident said, checking his work with his stethoscope.

Rich connected the ambu bag to the end of the airway tube and began ventilating the patient. Another resident entered and began firing away orders for medications. Nancy started preparing medicines, shooting the tops off the premixed syringes two at a time like she was playing tiddly winks. I grabbed my pen and became the official recorder, documenting all meds given since Tammy would never be able to reconstruct the code activities after the fact.

"Why didn't you call us sooner?" the resident asked Tammy as he injected medication directly into the man's heart with a four inch needle.

"I would have, but it was too dark to find the phone," Tammy quipped angrily.

The second resident whispered to him, "The electricity's been out for awhile, it's been hell up here."

"Sorry, Tammy, I didn't realize. His attending should have put him on a respirator when he sent him up here. Don't worry, I think this old guys gonna get lucky tonight."

By the time the supervisor arrived on the scene, we had already formed a cohesive, smoothly operating team. The patient's heart rhythm had returned to normal and the respirator had rapidly improved the patient's color. She made a few notes on her rounds sheet, insincerely offered her assistance, then left.

Eventually, we had a chance to pass report on to the night shift, who had already begun working with the other patients on the unit. The nurse taking over my assignment had worked in ICUs for several years in a variety of places.

"So what's the helmet on the woman in Bed 2 for?" was the first question she fired at me, before we had even sat down.

I explained the rationale, as described by Debbie, almost ten hours earlier.

"Oh. That makes sense. I've never seen that before."

"Neither had I," I admitted.

"That's why I love this job," she said, "I learn something new all the time."

As an inexperienced nurse, I had difficulty separating what I should have known from what I should not be expected to know already. I avoided asking what I perceived to be a "dumb" question out of fear of appearing incompetent, preferring to hide behind a facade of intelligence. This experienced nurse reminded me that questions are integral to insure competent practice and continual learning. I learned a very basic lesson that evening from her. It was always okay to ask.

By the time the dust had settled and I returned to say good night to Mrs. Dearborne and to thank her for her calming stories, she was fast asleep.

Eventually, so was I.

"He who trusts in himself is a fool.."

Proverbs 28:26

10

Private Lessons

Main Hospital had been a great place to start my career. A teaching hospital is ideal for learners. The spirit of inquiry is not only welcomed, it is applauded. So when my husband was transferred out of state, I looked forward to the new learning opportunities ahead. I decided that I wanted to stay within the ICU environment and accepted the only 7 a.m. to 3 p.m.intensive care unit position available in my new home town.

Community Hospital's facility was much newer and more modern than my previous one had been. The addition of windows throughout the unit made the whole place less frightening, despite the intensity and serious tones of the staff. I was apprehensive at first, until I realized how well my previous experience had prepared me. In fact, despite Main Hospital's antiquated environment, treatment wise it was actually much more advanced. This could have been a result of the close proximity to New York City or just because it was a teaching hospital. Things I had been doing for over a year at Main were just being introduced to the staff at Community.

Community Hospital was a small close knit institution. It was not unusual to find many family members employed in different departments or that people had known each other since childhood. I discovered, accompanied by glares, that I was not only the first new RN to have been hired to the day shift in five years, I was the only four year, baccalaureate nurse in the unit. Oblivious to the impact of these factors on my acceptance by the staff, I enthusiastically set out to practice nursing in the same manner that I had become accustomed: questioning, sharing ideas, and setting priorities based on patient's needs. When faced with totally different procedures than what I had been already taught, I wanted explanations. Often the rationale was sound and I had no problem relearning it the Community Hospital way. Sometimes the response was simply, "Because that's the way we always do it."

There were occasions where no rationale existed and my questions made them uncomfortable. Like their practice of assigning an aide as the sole care giver to an ICU patient. One day, around 2 p.m., the charge nurse asked me to chart on the aide's patient for the 7 - 3 shift.

"I can't chart on a patient I haven't even seen all day."

"But we all do it. It's your turn. What's the big deal?" was their response.

"I'll be glad to do a full assessment on her and make an entry for 2 p.m." I countered.

"You need to make it from 7 a.m.," the charge nurse insisted.

I thought about it.

"I'm sorry, but I can't do it. What if something had happened this morning that I was unaware of? My charting makes me responsible for her, and I can't accept that."

"She's been stable all day. Just write the note. Why do you have to question everything?"

"I'm sorry, but I can't."

The charge nurse huffed away to the office and was quickly joined by her cronies who apparently had been waiting in the wings. I remained at the desk and continued to chart. They returned a minute later.

"You have to chart Karen. It's part of your assignment on the sheet," the charge nurse restated smugly.

Another nurse showed me the sheet that now had "Charting 2B" written next to my name.

"That wasn't there this morning and you know it," I replied, feeling my insides begin to boil.

Another of the cronies said, "I saw it. Why would we make this up?"

I shook my head.

"This is wrong. Aides caring for ICU patients is wrong too. If these patients are sick enough to be placed in ICU by their doctors, they should be getting RN care."

"We've done this for years and no one has ever complained before," the charge nurse defended her turf, face and neck visibly reddened, voice raised. "Our aides provide competent and appropriate care. We never assign them to a situation they can't handle."

I hadn't meant for her to take this personally. I tried a different angle.

"Your aides are excellent. This is not about them. This is about charting and it's legal implications." I paused to gather my thoughts and decided it was best to lose this battle. "I'll write a full note for 2 p.m. today, but next time I want to know what other patient I am responsible for in the morning." I turned and left to avoid further confrontation.

As the ICU nursing staff grew cold and less approachable, I found a safe haven in the confines of my patient's rooms. As the months passed, I established positive relationships with support services; secretaries, respiratory therapists, laboratory phlebotomists, operating room nurses who came to assist with procedures, as well as student nurses. They became my friends and confidants, while the well established clique of staff nurses grew more distant.

One day the respiratory therapist assigned to the unit came to me.

"You've got to be careful Karen. They are really watching you." He was referring to the old guard.

"What do you mean?"

"I overheard them talking about you. They don't like you very much."

"I sensed that. I just stay away from them as much as I can."

"Look, you are an excellent nurse. If I were sick, I'd want you to take care of me. But they don't see it. They don't like you questioning them. I think they are jealous."

"Of what?"

"You're young. You're married. You already have your Bachelor's and they really resent that you are going for your Master's. Got the picture yet?"

"I wasn't sure."

"Basically, you can't say anything to them that would be right."

"What do you suggest?"

"Just watch your step. You have friends here if you need us!"

"Thanks."

Different staff members started showing up in my patient's rooms at odd times, checking my IV's, respiratory equipment settings and watching if my medications were precisely on time. No nurse functions at a one hundred percent rate of perfection every day. If you watch closely enough, you could make even Florence Nightingale look like Attila the Hun.

A couple of weeks after the silent inquisition had begun, a staff meeting was held, and I wasn't invited, despite being the sole agenda item. The head nurse found me in a patient's room to let me know the outcome of this meeting that I hadn't even known about... my IV's weren't always on time... the staff were complaining about how difficult I was to work with... the staff didn't like the way I questioned things.

There was more, I think. All I can remember was the tears and humiliation and false kindness of the head nurse who hadn't even the courtesy to meet with me in private while she destroyed my self-esteem. She left me sitting in a chair in my patient's room, dazed. The respiratory therapist comforted me after she left.

"That was a rotten thing to do to you."

He had been in the corner of the room and had overheard everything.

"I deserved it," I replied shamefully.

"No one deserves to be treated the way they've treated you."

I walked over to my patient bringing a cool washcloth for his perspiring forehead. As I held his hand, I counted the IV drops. I was right on time today. I chuckled. I stared numbly as the accordion pump of the respirator rose and fell, up and down, peacefully rhythmic. The EKG monitor bleeped in perfect synchrony. The noise steadily rose to a crescendo in my mind until it only echoed in the distance. I was a hundred miles away, in my old unit, surrounded by supportive peers, learning every day, loving my work.

I was blasted back to reality by the entrance of my patient's wife, here for her brief hourly visit. I answered her questions perfunctorily. Although I myself felt like a paper doll pinned at the joints, I offered my support and encouragement to her in her time of anticipatory grief. I made it through report, carefully avoiding eye contact with anyone else, and then drove home to where only my husband could glue me back together.

Getting to work from that day forward was a challenge. Getting out of bed is never easy at 5:3O a.m., but when you hate your job, it is tortuous. I called in sick as much as I dared. Eventually I surrendered. I left the ICU and accepted a float position. That means you go wherever the staff is short on a given day. You need to adapt to each floors peculiarity and take care of a wide variety of patient problems. The best part is that you can avoid the inter-staff bickering and backstabbing. Nobody cared if you spent all day in your patient's rooms. They didn't miss you. Heck, they didn't even know you.

I did a lot of soul searching and self-recrimination after what turned out to be my final ICU experience. For many years, I analyzed where I had gone wrong and wondered how I could have handled things better with the women on the unit. I harbored a feeling that perhaps, I really wasn't that good of a technical nurse. It would be two decades before I surreptitiously met the RN who replaced me on the same unit and found out that this old guard had done the same thing to her. She too needed the healing that moment provided for both of us.

Although the glitz and excitement of ICU nursing was gone, surprisingly, I didn't miss it as much as I thought I would. Floating allowed me to rediscover a meaningful and self-fulfilling part of nursing. My patients could talk again, and they needed me to be there to listen.

"He who listens to a life-giving rebuke
will be at home among the wise.
He who ignores discipline despises himself,
but whoever heeds correction gains understanding.
"

Proverbs 15:31-33

11

Floating Around

The line moved quickly in the nursing office that morning. When it was my turn, the secretary looked up at my nametag.

"Karen?" She read, and then checked her list. "Third floor."

"Haven't been there yet," I replied.

She made no response, but looked up and through me, waiting for me to move out of the way so she could see the next nametag.

"Have a nice day," I responded to her silence before I left. The line behind me was equally unfriendly. My smiles and hellos went unreciprocated. I shrugged it off to pre-coffee personalities.

The elevator was almost closed as I rounded the bend. I reached in to make the door reopen by triggering the safety catch in the closing door. It was a painless trick I learned living on the 14th floor of a college dorm serviced by only two elevators.

Several of the nurses gasped, thinking my hand was about to get squished. One dove frantically towards the "Open Door" button even though the doors were already reopening. I stepped in feeling proud of my cleverness.

"You could have lost your hand doing that!" one said angrily.

"No," I responded. "If you know just where to push in the door, it automatically opens."

"And if you miss?" she snapped.

"Wouldn't it be easier to wait for the next elevator?" asked another.

I was thinking, "but not as much fun", but decided to stay quiet in this elevator filled with grizzly faces. I reached over to press three, and then instead of joining the others in studying the floor numbers above the door, I faced them all and smiled. Fortunately, no one from the elevator exited with me on the 3rd floor.

Although each Community hospital unit had an identical floor plan, there were distinct variations in how each operated. I spotted the space designated for report and took a seat next to the woman preparing to receive the morning update.

"Who are you?" she asked.

"Karen, I'm a float. This is my first time on 3."

The woman without a nametag looked me over with her eyes. Spotting the stethoscope around my neck she asked, "Are you new here?"

Back in those days, only critical care nurses and students wore their stethoscopes like necklaces.

"Been at Community about a year. Mostly in ICU. I've been floating a few months but this is my first time on 3."

"Very nice," she replied sounding bored. "Did you see your morning assignment?"

"No, where is it?"

"At the station." The woman turned from me and motioned to the night nurse to begin report.

I remained in my seat, listening and wondering when the other nurses would arrive to listen to report. Before the second patient report began, the woman turned back to me and said, "I said, your assignment is at the desk."

"What about report?" I asked innocently.

"The staff don't listen to report. They do their morning assignments."

"Can't I stay and listen?"

"No. I'll tell you what you need to know."

The night nurse waited impatiently as I gathered my pens and paper to leave, bewildered and embarrassed. After a brief pause, I heard the reporting resume.

I walked out to the station and located the assignment. Aides, LPNs, and RNs were all scattering to complete their morning tasks. In this Functional Method of nursing, tasks, like blood pressures, filling ice water, and counting narcotics, were assigned to workers as opposed to patient's being assigned to care givers. While cost effective, it lacks a sense of personalized attention. On paper, having all staff responsible for all patients, looks good. But receiving care from ten different caregivers during a single shift can be disconcerting, fragmented and impersonal. Elderly patients who are disoriented from the displacement into the hospital to begin with can get more confused with the parade of changing faces.

I completed my morning tasks, greeting each patient by name and visiting cheerily, wrongly assuming that I would return later to provide care. Noting a gathering of staff at the nurses' station, I returned to find that I was assigned to eight beds; two four-bed rooms on the opposite end of the hall I had just been. One bed was empty, but an admission was expected. I was handed an assignment sheet that contained the patient's last name, room number, and specific care required.

"Check incision," I read. "Where's the incision?" I asked the woman who had taken report.

She looked at my sheet and pointed to the letters P.O.

"He's post op," she said with a sigh, then walked away.

"What are my patient's diagnoses," I asked, talking to no one in particular.

"You don't need them. We work from these sheets all the time," a nurse standing within earshot responded. Let me see who you've got."

I handed her my sheet.

"You've got the girls, pointing to the bottom four names. They can be a handful. They all had strokes or something. They are all completes. The men across the hall are nice. I had them yesterday. My name is Leesa. Call me if you need a hand. I'm on meds on that side."

"Thanks." Although her information lacked depth, I was grateful for a friendly response.

I gathered my linen in anticipation of a long morning of hygiene focused care. The men looked quiet, so I began in the ladies room. The woman in Bed A was non-communicative and immobile. Her facial drooping confirmed the stroke diagnosis. The lady in Bed B was alert but very confused. She had no other obvious symptoms of a stroke and was able to help with her own bath. The lady in Bed C told me she was on bedrest because of a fractured pelvis. The lady in Bed D needed a dressing change to her lower leg. She asked me for the bedpan and from my sheet I saw that she was also on bed-rest, but otherwise I had no clue to her underlying problems.

As I washed my hands at the sink, I looked up at my image in the mirror. Instead of the usual make-up check, my eyes became fixed on my nametag. The initials "R.N." glared at me like an illuminated billboard, a reminder of the level of care I was educated to provide. Today, with inadequate data on my patients, I was just an overpaid nurses' aide and it was making me quite uncomfortable. I started back to the nurses' station when Leesa called me.

"Karen? Your light is on in 15."

"Thanks." I hesitated for a minute, debating if I really wanted to continue my RN charade. As usual, patient comfort won.

"You rang?" I said, entering the room.

The man in Bed C needed his urinal emptied. When I returned the emptied urinal to his bed-stand, the man in Bed C asked, "Will I be getting out of bed today?"

Checking my sheet I saw that Mr. Dungston was the mystery post-op man.

"Yes. How about after breakfast today?"

"Oh, do I get breakfast today?"

"Ummm.." I looked at my sheet again. No diets were listed. "Let me double check. How's the incision?"

"Feels okay. Want to see?" he asked, pulling up his gown.

Following his lead, I helped the gown up to reveal a nicely healing abdominal incision.

"Will I have any restrictions on my diet when I get home?" he asked.

"That's up to the doctor." Safe answer.

"How about activity restrictions?"

"After any abdominal surgery there are restrictions," I answered feeling blinded by my lack of knowledge. "Mr. Dungston, can you excuse me a minute? I left another patient on a bedpan." It was a lie, but I had to get out of there before he asked me anything else. Mr. Dungston and my other patients deserved more.

I went straight to the nurses' station. Spotting the kardex, I began to flip through, looking for my first patient. The woman who took report got up from her chair and stood next to me. This time she was wearing her R.N. nametag.

"Is there something you need?"

"I need a little more information on my patients."

"Like what, specifically?"

"I need a diet," I began.

"They are on this clipboard over here," she said picking up the kardex and walking me to a list hanging on a pillar.

"Okay, but I still want to check the kardex on my other patients."

"The information is on your sheet already. The secretary needs the kardex now for orders."

"Isn't it a nursing kardex?" I asked, treading in deep waters.

"It isn't available right now," she said walking away with it tucked under her arm.

Frustrated, but not out of ideas, I went to the chart rack and pulled Mr. Dungston's chart. Skimming through the physician's note I discovered that he had a cholecystectomy (gall bladder removal) the previous day. If he had bowel sounds today, we would be giving him a jello and tea breakfast. It turned out he had a long history of gall stones and also respiratory problems. I would need to add some vigorous respiratory exercises to the day's agenda to prevent post-op pneumonia. I would get Respiratory Therapy to send me a breathing "toy" to encourage deep breaths. He had been hospitalized last June for a blood clot in his leg. I would need to initiate some appropriate nursing measures for that as well.

My confused lady in Bed B was admitted because she had been found in her apartment barely conscious and extremely dehydrated. She would not be going back home. Arrangements to place her in a nursing home were underway. Although this was a common reason for hospitalization, it is psychologically devastating to the person in the bed, requiring patience and a willing ear.

The lady in Bed A with the stroke had been in her current vegetative state for over six months now. She was gradually deteriorating and had been unresponsive to all therapies.

The woman with the leg dressing had cellulitis, a potentially serious skin infection. Her wound was the result of insufficient venous drainage. This was her second hospitalization for the wound this year. I decided to find out more about what she did at home to care for herself. I remembered seeing a knee high stocking held up with a rubber band on the other leg. This was clearly a good teaching opportunity.

The lady with the pelvic fracture had just been diagnosed with bone cancer. The oncologist had come yesterday and told her that a round of chemotherapy and radiation would buy her time. My priorities for care on this woman were now totally different.

The other two men were both post-op from prostate surgery. One would be going home today, so he would need some post-op/discharge teaching early this morning. The other man had passed some large blood clots yesterday and he needed to be monitored. My sheet from H. Langley R.N. included, "P.O., Foley catheter, I and O." Nothing about blood clots.

While I had been skimming these charts, a ten-minute investment of time, several nurses and doctors looked at me strangely.

"What's she doing?" I overheard one nurse ask H. Langley R.N.

"She didn't like my sheets," she snapped.

I was folding up my sheet, now cluttered with personal notes, when H. Langley said, "Your lights are on Karen."

"Thanks, be right there," breathing a sigh of relief, happy to be wearing RN shoes again.

I avoided working on the 3rd floor from then on whenever possible, but when I did, my day always began in the chart rack. Inevitably some nurse would ask me what I was doing.

"Oh, it's habit, I'd respond," belittling its' value in attempt to not stand out.

"Boy it must be nice to have that kind of time," they would reply on their way to get their morning coffee and cup of gossip.

Tension and stress were packaged and expressed in different ways on each unit that I floated to. Some groups of staff never spoke to one another. Others ganged up against the management on any issue. Some complained endlessly about their workload. A few began each day checking the classified ads. There were floors with demanding, chronically ill elderly with surprisingly content staff and floors with challenging or pleasant younger adult patients with miserable staff. Without question, the personality of the nurse manager set the tone for the unit. I had learned a valuable lesson in the ICU and despite the occasionally volatile nature of working with many hormonally dominant females, I got along with my fellow staff nurses on the general floors at Community.

It was nearing the end of a long day when I saw a doctor duck into Mr. Graves room. Mr. Graves was a 76 year old gentleman in for multiple tests. We had a pleasant conversation earlier in the day. He was retired. His wife died several years ago of cancer. His children were grown with kids of their own and lived out of the area. He lived in his own apartment and had several buddies living nearby with whom he regularly socialized. I entered the room in time to hear Dr. Diamond, well known for his caustic bedside manner, begin.

"Mr. Graves, I've reviewed your tests and it's clear that you have widespread cancer of your bladder and prostate," he continued on without pausing, "so I'm going to schedule you for surgery tomorrow and we will start chemotherapy by the end of this week or the beginning of the next."

Mr. Graves was in obvious shock. Tears began to well up in his eyes. I walked to his side, took his hand and put my other hand on his shoulder.

"Are you sure?" Mr. Graves asked.

"Mr. Graves," Dr. Diamond sighed, revealing an annoyance at having been questioned, "You've been peeing blood for weeks. You must have known that there was a problem."

"How much time do I have?"

"Your cancer is very advanced. A couple of months, maybe."

"I want to go home first," he said, tears dripping off his cheek.

"That's out of the question, Mr. Graves."

"I want to go home for just a day or two to get my affairs in order while I know I can still get around. I don't want my children to have to deal with all of my things. I went through this when my wife got sick."

It sounded reasonable to me.

"Absolutely not," the doctor responded.

"Doctor, I promise I will come back. Today is Monday. I'll come back, let's say, Thursday and then I'm all yours. Surely two days can't make that much of a difference at this point."

"I can't agree to that." Dr. Diamond held firm.

"How long will it be before I'm able to go home?"

"Probably several weeks. But I can't guarantee. You may never be able to."

Mr. Graves began to openly weep.

"It's my body. I want to go home."

"You are my patient and I will not sign you out," Dr. Diamond's voice began to rise as the patient's whimpering increasingly agitated him.

"Please doctor, I'm not asking for much," he begged between sobs.

"Calm yourself down, Mr. Graves. You are a grown man."

Dr. Diamond's approach was in stark contrast to the handholding soft tone I had grown accustomed to seeing other physicians use in these situations. I admired how even the perpetually gruff, hyper-focused, no-nonsense physicians melted into compassionate putty at the bedside of a patient when they had to deliver bad news. This man was different. I had never been witness to such a degrading and insensitive interchange. I could no longer remain silent.

"Doctor, since Mr. Graves is able to get around on his own right now, perhaps a day or two at home makes sense," I suggested gently.

"This is my patient. I know what I am doing. He's just not rational right now."

I stood up and spoke quietly to Dr. Diamond. "Perhaps if you leave, I can get him calmed down."

"How dare you ask me to leave? Who do you think you are?"

"I'm just trying to help," I said.

"This is none of your business," he snapped. "If you want to help, go get 5 mg of Valium for Mr. Graves, IM stat."

I didn't move. I was afraid to leave the trembling patient alone with this fury filled physician.

"Two days.. I just want to go home for two days," Mr. Graves cried.

I held tight to his hand. His eyes looked to me imploringly.

"I know," I said quietly.

Dr. Diamond spoke harshly, "I have had enough of this.

Nurse, I gave you a direct order to get a shot of Valium for Mr. Graves. NOW!"

"The only one who needs a Valium around here is you!" I blurted impulsively.

"Get out of here," Dr. Diamond spoke forcefully, his eyes sternly focused on my face.

"I refuse to leave my patient alone with you. You are out of control, doctor."

"This is unbelievable," the doctor said as he turned on his heels and charged out of the room.

I stayed with Mr. Graves and gradually his sobbing slowed as he regained his composure. When the head nurse appeared with a syringe in her hand, I knew I was in trouble.

"Dr. Diamond wants Mr. Graves to have a shot of Valium," she said.

"I know. But he's much calmer now."

Mr. Graves spoke, "Let her give me the shot. It can't hurt." He squeezed my hand. "Thank you for sticking up for me."

"I'm not done yet, Mr. Graves," I winked. "I'll go talk with him."

Dr. Diamond was seated at the desk scribbling notes in a chart. He looked up as I entered the station and walked over to me.

"I want to get your name," he said in a loud bellowing voice. Reading my nametag aloud he said, "Karen Smith, RN. You call yourself a nurse? I have never seen such a display of disregard for a physician in all my years of practice. You don't deserve to call yourself an RN."

The bustling activity in the station had come to a complete halt as Dr. Diamond's booming voice echoed.

"Dr. Diamond, I apologize. My comment about the Valium was out of line."

"You're damn right it was out of line. You obviously don't know whom you are dealing with. I bring a lot of patients to this hospital. I could have you fired. You don't deserve to wear that uniform. You are a terrible nurse."

My voice rose in response, "I will not stand here and allow you slander my nursing ability."

"You want to sue me? I could bring you up for professional

misconduct."

"Doctor, I may have been out of line with my comment to you, but you were out of line with the patient. Thank God I was in there. I have never been witness to such an abominable and insensitive treatment of a patient."

"How dare you insult me like that? He is my patient and I will talk to him any way I like."

Mustering maximum control, I spoke softly in attempt to defuse this near hostile confrontation.

"All Mr. Graves wanted was to go home for two days."

"If he goes home, he won't come back. He waited three weeks to come this time."

"But he did come in, and he would come back. That man is devastated in there."

"That is why, <u>Nurse</u> Smith, that I ordered the Valium."

"He didn't need Valium, he needed empathy."

"I do this all the time. I know what I am doing. The patient will deal with it just fine. I don't need to answer to a nurse, especially one who doesn't know her place."

"My place is to serve as a patient advocate. When you lost control, it was my place to support the patient, which is what I did."

"It was your place to support the physician. What kind of school did you go to?"

"A Baccalaureate program."

He huffed.

"Did they teach you it was okay to insult physicians there?"

"Apparently we have a difference of opinion as to the role of a nurse that won't be resolved here. More importantly, it won't resolve Mr. Graves need, and right to go home."

"As far as I'm concerned, there are no issues to resolve. He is my patient. He stays. You are supposed to be the nurse, but you apparently don't know who your boss is. I'm appalled at your lack of professionalism. I don't know how you ever got hired."

"I can't understand why you keep attacking me personally. This shouldn't be about me and you, Dr. Diamond. This should be about what is best for the patient."

"Yes, this IS about you and me. And this is not over. I am going to report you to the Director of Nursing. I will not tolerate such subordination."

"Go ahead and report me. I will have no difficulty defending my behavior."

The head nurse interrupted at this point with a quiet voice. "Dr. Diamond, I can't have you two continuing this in the nurses' station. There are visitors around. You are welcome to use my office."

"I'm done anyway," he said. He looked at me and spoke sternly, "I do not want you to get near my patient's again, for absolutely any reason." Turning back to the head nurse he said firmly, "Do I make myself clear?"

"Yes, Dr. Diamond," she replied.

It was powerless moments like this when my choice to be "just" a nurse haunted me the most.

Although I was on that floor again the next day, my assignment was changed. I made one feeble attempt to see Mr. Graves, but was quickly thwarted by the medicine nurse on that side of the hall. Even though Dr. Diamond was not well liked by the staff nurses, as a float nurse, I was a nobody who had created unsolicited havoc for their floor.

Dr. Diamond followed through on his threat as I suspected he would. The Director of Nursing met with me and the Head Nurse the next afternoon. After hearing both sides of the story and being well aware of Dr. Diamond's bedside reputation, she decided that a mutual reprimand was in order.

"We don't like to discourage nurses from becoming patient advocates," she began with a serious tone. "Dr. Diamond is rarely challenged at this institution and perhaps from what you tell us, it was justified in this circumstance. However, loud arguments in a nursing station are never appropriate and I cannot condone these behaviors. I can assure you that Dr. Diamond has been told that you are a highly qualified and skilled nurse and that we have no intentions of firing you over this incident. But it is within his right to ask that you no longer care for his patients. I hope that you will be professional in any future dealings with him."

"What about Mr. Graves?" I asked.

"He is his patient and no longer your concern. I've heard his surgery went well. Stay away Karen. It's not worth it."

"I hate to think that Dr. Diamond is treating others the way he treated Mr. Graves."

"I've asked the Medical Director to discuss his handling of this incident with Dr. Diamond. Perhaps some good will come of it."

The head nurse joined in, "You weren't the first one to notice Dr. Diamond's bedside manner, but you were the first to take him on for it."

"I'd do it again too."

"We know. That's why we are asking you to stay clear of him."

"I'll behave. I promise," I said crossing my fingers under the desk like a kid promising the impossible to her teacher.

Most physicians are devoted servants to their profession who appreciate the input that the eyes and ears of nurses have to offer to the health care team. Fortunately, there are only a few "Dr. Diamonds" to contend with along the way. Unfortunately, as a nurse, physicians rule the roost. As a nurse you win some and lose some. If your intentions are good, it's worth the fight. The wounds of the battle always heal, especially if you "float" away.

Be completely humble and gentle; be patient, bearing with one another in love. Make every effort to keep the unity of the spirit through the bond of peace.

Ephesians 4: 2-3

12

Beyond the Shadow of a Wrinkle

Tired of floating and working random shifts, I left Community Hospital to work full-time days at a nearby nursing home. I had gone from super high tech to medium tech to low tech and surprised myself to find a tremendously rewarding experience. The nursing home patients, referred to as "residents", sucked up love and attention like a dry sponge and blossomed in front of your eyes.

Like all nursing homes, this one came complete with the standard sensory images: residents lining the hallways in wheelchairs; occasional gagging whiffs of stale urine; episodic shouts or cries, generally indiscernible, but at times profanity appropriate only for a football locker room. Yet each resident endeared themselves to me by their unique character or peculiarities when you looked beyond their wrinkles.

"There goes Dorothy again."

The aide moved towards a woman slumped to the side in the corner wheelchair post. Dorothy, a stroke patient, spoke only profanity.

"Shit, shit, shit, shit, shit.."

This had nothing to do with her need to go to the bathroom. It was not a code word. We learned to tell what she wanted not by her selection of words, but by the tone and urgency in her voice. If you tried to get Dorothy to do something she didn't want to do, she would offer up a line that might make a truck driver blush.

Dorothy was a retired schoolteacher with a small petite frame that suggested a life of church suppers and needlepoint. This was her twisted fate, the result of a damaged pre-frontal cortex. We did our best to make sure she was content during family visiting hours to prevent eyebrow-raising episodes.

Sam the Weatherman took his post next to the Number One Elevator at 6 a.m. daily to await the arrival of his newspaper. Sam greeted everyone that entered the unit throughout the day and would verify the accuracy of the weather report.

"Supposed to rain this morning," he could be heard saying to a passerby.

"Hasn't started yet, Sam," the passerby responded.

Minutes later the elevator door opened again.

"Supposed to rain today," he offered once again.

"Hope not," the aide said as she walked past, "I didn't bring my umbrella."

"Eighty percent chance by midday. Storms coming from the Southeast today."

"Is that so. Uh huh," said another.

Sam looked down into his paper disappointed.

Another aide, who had paused outside the elevator to reposition her hold on her bags, stopped and squatted down next to Sam.

"I didn't hear the weather yet Sam. How's it look for this afternoon?"

Sam's face immediately lit up.

"Supposed to have rain this morning, but clearing by late afternoon!"

"Hear anything about tomorrow yet?"

"Looks good through Friday!"

"I'm glad I can count on you to know Sam, I always forget to check."

"They don't call me Sam the Weatherman for nothing!"

"Gotta go Sam," the aide stood up, waved good-bye, "I'll see you later."

"Okay." Sam replied as his gaze followed the aide to the locker room behind the nurses station. A new level of alertness was clearly evident on his face. Ready, willing, and eager to offer service to all.

Mabel Rose owned the position opposite Sam at the elevator. Hall positions had to be learned and respected by all caregivers. It was not unusual to have territorial disputes if an unknowing aide positioned a less alert resident in someone else's spot. Residents who claimed themselves incapable of pushing their own wheelchair into the dining room would find the strength to push another resident out of their spot, no matter how long it took, or where the other resident wound up. Bickering among the residents often led to some pretty nasty fights.

Mabel and Rose had become friends. They would look out for each other by calling the nurse for assistance if the other needed help.

"Nurse, Rose needs to be pulled up," Mabel would call.

They weren't roommates, although they could have been if they had wanted to. One day, Mabel wasn't feeling too well so when she wheeled herself down the hall and around the corner to the elevators and saw Rose in her spot she lost it.

"You're in my spot!" Mabel shouted.

"You don't own this!" Rose countered, although had the positions been reversed, she would have been just as angry.

"I sit there every day and you know it."

"Big deal."

Mabel maneuvered her wheelchair around for the kill, butting the side of Rose's.

"What are you trying to do, kill me? I'm getting pretty tired of you pushing me around here every day," Rose shouted.

Rose shoved Mabel's wheelchair back with her foot, albeit clumsily.

"I'm tired of listening to you complaining and whining," Mabel changed to a mimicking tone of voice, "Ohh my legs, my legs."

"You witch! You don't know half the pain I've lived with every day for twenty years."

Sam watched with obvious enjoyment at this highlight of his day. Feigning anger he chirped in, "You two nags, stop flapping your jaws so loud. A man can't find his peace in this place!"

By now, Mabel had maneuvered herself close enough to grab the sidearm of Rose's wheelchair and visa versa. They had an armlock deadlock, and with grits on their faces, both were determined to hang on.

"You're going to have a heart attack if you don't let go," Mabel said.

"You're going to have a stroke first," Rose countered as they glared into each other's eyes.

They began to bat at each other with their free arms.

As entertaining as this had become, I decided the ladies had let off enough steam for one day and moved in to act as arbitrator. It took two of us, myself and an aide, to pry their grasps loose from each other.

"Come on you two, you're friends."

We positioned them in their own "spots" and I sent the aide to get some juice. Since the free arm batting hadn't stopped, I placed myself in between them, catching a few harmless swipes in my side as I did so. The arrival of the cranberry juice distracted the women and they eventually settled for a few nasty exchanges as they drank the magic healing potion. An hour later, no one would have known there had been a problem.

"Nurse, nurse, Rose needs help, she's sliding out of her chair," Mabel called.

"We're coming Mabel. Don't worry, she's not going to fall."

"Yeah, this time. One of these days I'm not going to be here to warn you girls in time."

"Mabel, you're going to outlive us all," said the aide as she kissed her on the cheek.

Jack was the ladies man on the unit. He positioned himself where the action was and was welcomed wherever he went. The ladies giggled like schoolgirls as he swooned them on his daily rounds. He made eyes at all the female staff and would linger longer than necessary on the girl's shoulders when he was being transferred between his wheelchair and his bed. Residents often put their hands around your waist for support, but Jack managed a suggestive grip. We all learned to turn, slip away, and keep him from falling in one easy maneuver.

"How about a kiss, baby. You'd make an old man so happy."

"Jack, you're cute, but I'm married," I'd say, moving on to the business at hand.

Although he made us uncomfortable at times, he had his endearing qualities. You had to respect such a relentless libido in an 87 year old man. Yes, it was sexual harassment, but he didn't know it. It had been his way for a lifetime. Harsher correction for his behavior would have been more destructive to him than he ever could be to us.

Josie was a 71 year old woman transferred to us from Community Hospital. She "survived" a massive stroke. She was unable to move her right side at all and it had assumed a fetal like position. It was impossible to straighten it without triggering obvious intense pain. Her left side moved spontaneously, but not purposefully. She could not speak. Her eyes stared aimlessly towards the wall she faced. She was able to eat and swallow if fed, but unable to wipe drool from her own chin.

Josie's room was filled with pictures... Josie's family reunion from the last Fourth of July. Pictures of Josie's 18 grandchildren and pictures drawn by tiny hands signed "Love You Nana" or "We Miss You". Pictures of a vibrant Josie, arm in arm with her girlfriends, suntanned and all ready to tee off. There was even a picture of her on stage dressed as a dancer from years before. Josie had probably attended college in her fifties as one picture showed her dressed in a cap and gown, proudly displaying her diploma, cheered by her daughters and sons.

Josie wasn't looking at these pictures. We were. Josie could never become just a "body" in the bed to us caregivers surrounded by such a vivid portrayal of her life. Even though each floor had a dozen Josies, each were unique.

Enter the "Not-Too-Verbals". A group of men and women who sat quietly in the dayroom at their meal tables all day. Breakfast would come and go. Lunch would come and go. They would be taken to their rooms in the afternoon for a nap, and then wheeled back in time for dinner to come and go.

Mr. Thomas, Adele, and Bessie only moved when they needed to scratch a body part or shift their weight off their bottom. Frieda Johnson would bend and pick up dropped napkins from the floor then slowly shred them on her lap. Beatrice and Wanda would ask for the meal tables that gave them the best view of the television, then remain glued to whatever channel played all day long.

These men and women seemed content to sit and watch others. Perhaps they had done that all of their lives. Perhaps they chose to turn off their minds rather than confront the reality of their confinement due to their fading physical abilities. Keeping the Not-Too-Verbals clean and fed was tedious at times, but easily achieved. Reaching them was a challenge. The nursing home did a marvelous job providing a myriad of social activities for the residents. Bingo and other games, crafts, guests from community groups doing all kinds of different things, and movies to name a few.

One of my favorites was a sing-a-long. To an outsider, the level of resident participation would have appeared meager and unenthusiastic. But I saw something much different. Adele mouthed the words of one familiar old tune and Bessie's eyes became teary during a love song. Frieda sang along in a weak, crackly voice and never missed a word. Mr. Thompson held the words in his hands, though never uttering a sound, followed along in silence. Beatrice tapped her fingers, almost to the beat of the music. Wanda sang the choruses and the first line or so of each verse, occasionally blurting out a word, her eyes closed the whole time. Others in the room watched on, expressionless. I never knew what memories were sparked or what they were thinking of at times like this. I only knew that music was a powerful tool in reaching their minds.

Getting them to move around and use their bodies was more difficult. I found the most powerful tool to get them to participate in physical exercise was trickery. When you asked them to raise their arms the response was anemic. Blow up a plastic glove like a balloon and even the weakest resident joined in a high reaching game of table volleyball, even if it was just to swat an incoming serve away from their face. Another effective exercise was to place cookies on a plate that required a very long reach across the table. There is sometimes a fine line between being mean and being effective.

My role as RN in the nursing home was to act as the unit Charge Nurse, which meant a day of total paperwork, or to act as Medication or Treatment Nurse. The aides were responsible to wash and dress the patients then change the linens.

Providing care to residents was by nature monotonous. They got the same medications everyday at the same time. The residents preferred no variations in their routines for daily bathing, dressing, and toileting. But thanks to their personal idiosyncrasies, it was possible to find humor and satisfaction even in the daily monotony.

On occasions I took an "aides" assignment. The pace was exhausting and the amount of lifting, bending, reaching, and pulling strained even the most physically fit of us. Depending on the staffing, an aide might have as many as ten patients to care for in a day. To do this very well, and at a nice pace, each patient would need a full hour of personal attention a day. With eight hour shifts and ten patients, minus lunch, coffee breaks, and feeding hours, the math doesn't work out that nicely. It was especially frustrating when these elderly patients, preferring a slower pace to match their own cerebral and physical speeds, would find ways to make you slow down.

"Mrs. Tanner, your bath is done now. Let me get your chair," I offered, moving towards the door.

"Would you hand me my comb again?"

"Sure," I said, handing her the comb on the bedside stand.

"Not that one. I want the pink one that's in the dresser."

I looked in the dresser and rummaged around a bit.

"No sign of a pink comb Mrs. Tanner."

"Try the other drawer."

This went on till I searched six drawers, a closet, and her purse.

"Mrs. Tanner, I can't find it anywhere."

"I'll have to get my daughter to find it when she comes. Bring me that powder," pointing as she spoke.

I brought a perfumed powder that was on the dresser and sat it on her lap. She opened it painstakingly slowly.

"Can I help you with that?"

"Oh no, I can manage quite well thank you."

Finally opened, she took a sniff, leaving a white residue on the tip of her nose.

"This isn't the right one. My daughter-in-law gave me this cheap stuff. Makes me smell like a funeral parlor. She probably got it on sale somewhere." Then with a whisper added, "She's a cheap one if you know what I mean. Grab that blue one."

I brought the other powder over, opening it before I handed it to her this time.

"It's already open Mrs. Tanner."

Mrs. Tanner, with hand shaking, took the blue powder and slowly closed the top then slowly opened it again, either to check my intelligence or her abilities. Eventually she was powdered. She had me find three other things for her lap and soon we were headed out the door. My fourth patient for the day was almost done.

"Nurse, wait a minute."

"Yes Mrs. Tanner?" I said, feigning enthusiasm.

"I think I better go to the bathroom before we leave."

"Of course, Mrs. Tanner."

These elderly patients didn't deliberately drive us crazy. Patients like Mrs. Tanner were just lonely and once they got our attention, they didn't want to let go. Watching my own parents suffer from the aftermaths of strokes, I realize now how scary it is to be immobilized. Dependency is neither desired nor natural. When someone is unable to meet their own basic needs without a helping hand, it is a huge emotional burden for them to adapt to.

They sit and wonder… The next time I sneeze, will I be able to reach the tissue I knocked on the floor? Or will I have to wipe my nose with my sleeve again? How long will I need to sit in this wet diaper that I am wearing today, not because I'm incontinent, but because it is so labor intensive to get me on the toilet?

Working with the elderly is a special calling. Not just because it is hard physical labor. Not just because elderly patients tend to have multiple chronic illnesses that all need attention. Not just because patients are often hard of hearing and tend to move and process things very slowly. Working with elderly is difficult because you are working with your future staring you in the face every day. As a care giver, it is hard to not ask yourself, "If I am blessed with longevity, what curse will I bear, what thorn will be in my side?"

Will I swear like Dorothy? Will I be fixated on the weather like Sam? Will I have a friend like Mabel or Rose to watch out for me but need to occasionally bicker with to prove I've still got spunk? Will I cross moral boundaries like Jack? Will my useless body be maintained in the shadow of my prior existence like

Josie? Will my daily routine be reduced to hygiene and meals like the "Not-Too-Verbals?" Will I be so lonely and bored that I will harass my caregivers with nonsense requests like Mrs. Tanner?

Will people know my name or even care about who I was and what I accomplished before I became the wrinkled woman in room 4A with the light on?

It's hard to describe the deep feeling of self-satisfaction that comes from providing a service to someone that is both needy and appreciative. This is the priceless take home bonus of working with geriatrics.

"Do not lose heart
though outwardly we are wasting away,
yet inwardly we are being renewed day by day.
For our light and momentary troubles are achieving
for us an eternal glory that far outweighs them all.
So we fix our eyes not on what is seen,
but on what is unseen.
For what is seen is temporary,
but what is unseen is eternal."

2 Corinthians 4:16

13

Lessons of the Law

"You have the right to remain silent. You have the right to obtain and have an attorney present. What you say can and will be used against you in a court of law.."

My stomach dropped to my toes! After having worked for years in fast paced, high risk areas without a legal hitch, it was my ironic fate to tangle with the law while employed in a nursing home. How did I ever get myself in this mess?

There was a rapid turnover of aide personnel in the nursing home due to the heavy workload and the low pay. The hiring policies were lenient and at times it seemed based only on the existence of warm blood as evidenced by a typical morning conversation among the staff.

"Good weekend off?" Andrea, one of the aides, asked me.

"Yeah, nothing exciting. Cut the lawn, watched some movies. How about you?"

"Went to a wild party Saturday! There must have been fifty of us in the kitchen at one point. It was great."

"Sounds like fun."

"It wasn't fun once my ex got there. Boy did he get p.. off when he saw me there with Buzz, my new boyfriend. I just kept kissing Buzz on the cheek till he went nuts. My ex started throwing s.. all over the place and broke a lamp."

"How terrible."

"No, it was great. Buzz and three of his buddies picked him up and tossed him out into the street on his a... Then I ran out and grinded my spike heel right into his hand. It was awesome."

"Ohhh. I'll bet," trying hard to pretend it sounded like fun to me too.

Others had joined us, so I slipped away. From the crowds' response, there was more to the story, but I wasn't quite sure I could give the responses of support she had in mind. I quickly found something else to keep me busy. While I found it important to maintain good relationships with all the aides, it wasn't necessary to pretend I was their best buddy.

Several weeks later, I took a break from my paperwork to give the aides a hand. I walked down the hall till I found a room of unmade beds. I was halfway through making the bed when Dawn and Rebecca joined me.

"Wow, this is a treat," Rebecca said.

"You don't have to do this," Dawn added.

"I don't mind," I said as I continued with the top sheets.

The two aides pitched in to help.

"Some of the nurses wouldn't get caught dead helping us," Rebecca said.

"You should tell her what you told me," Dawn said to Rebecca. "You can trust her."

My curiosity was peaked.

"Tell me what?"

Rebecca looked troubled. She hesitated, and then tested the waters.

"I saw something the other day. I don't know what to do about it."

"Saw something?"

"My husband told me to keep my mouth shut. I need this job."

I waited as she finished the bed then went to the door and closed it.

"I saw someone hit a patient."

"Are you sure?"

"I was in the doorway. I had come because I heard her yelling at a patient. Apparently the resident was giving her a hard time about getting dressed." Rebecca paused and swallowed hard. "Just as I got there, I saw her swing hard and slap the poor woman."

"Who was it?" I asked as gently as I could.

Rebecca's eyes averted mine. "I don't know if I want to say," again a long pause.

"This girl once threatened someone in the parking lot that

she'd beat them up if they reported her.

Dawn joined in, "She broke a woman's arm last year. They said it was an accident."

"Was it Andrea?" I guessed the one who attacked her ex.

"Yes."

"You're doing the right thing Rebecca. This can't go on. I don't know what to do, but I promise that I'll follow through. Thanks for trusting me."

I had no clue what to do with this second hand story, so I immediately went and found Sara, my Head Nurse. She recommended that we speak with the Nursing Director immediately. After the Nursing Director heard the story, she assured us that we had done the right thing to come to her.

"We will begin an immediate in-house investigation of this. Please send Rebecca down so that we can talk with her." the Director asked.

When we got upstairs, Dawn told us that Rebecca had called her husband after we had spoken and he had told her to pack her stuff and wait for him to pick her up at the back door. I ran back downstairs to find her, but she was gone. The Director of Nursing told us not to worry. They would contact her at home.

The next day, a Friday, we found out that Rebecca had not answered her phone all evening. It wasn't until late in the afternoon that Rebecca did answer, apparently when her husband stepped out. She repeated the same story to the Director and then gave her resignation, effective immediately. The Director assured us that an in-house investigation had begun and that we would be kept informed.

"Your part is done. Now go home and enjoy your weekend," she said smiling.

Monday we were informed that the Director was going to place a call to the Patient Abuse Hotline, an information line just recently established by the State Health Department.

Tuesday afternoon, shortly after report, Sara and I were called down to the Director's office. No one was smiling. Several men, dressed in suits, looking very official, awaited our arrival. I was asked to wait in the outer office while Mary was taken in to an adjoining room. Twenty minutes later Sara emerged, looking frazzled and pale. Before she could say anything, my name was called.

I entered the conference room that was noticeably devoid of the usual gaiety. Seated at the table were two state officials and several administrators of the nursing home. As I sat down at the table the state investigator began.

"You have the right to remain silent..."

Feeling like a criminal, yet knowing I had done nothing wrong, I relaxed a little assuming this was just part of the routine for data collection.

"How long have you been employed here at this nursing home?"

"About seven months."

"What is your job title here?"

"Staff RN."

"Are you aware of the Patient Abuse Reporting Law?"

"I know that I'm supposed to report abuse."

"Just yes or no please, Mrs. Smith."

"Yes."

"What is your understanding of that law?"

"If I see abuse, I must report it to someone."

"Would you describe the events of last Thursday to us?"

I told my story to the expressionless people at the table. The two state investigators wrote notes and occasionally nodded, though it was neither approval nor disapproval. When I finished, the questioning resumed.

"When the aide had told you about the patient being hit, why didn't you call the patient abuse hotline?"'

"I thought it was my responsibility to report it to my supervisor, which I did, immediately."

"When your supervisor had not called the hotline by the next day, why didn't you call the hotline at that time?"

"It was my understanding that the nursing home was conducting an in-house investigation of the incident."

"When the state had not been notified by Monday morning, why didn't you call the hotline at that time?"

"I was under the understanding that the nursing home was planning to notify the state that day."

"Did anyone from the nursing home advise you to call the Patient Abuse Hotline?"

"No."

"Did anyone from the nursing home prevent you from calling the Patient Abuse Hotline?"

"No."

"Are you aware that under the Patient Reporting of Abuse Act, you were under obligation to report this incident to the State at the time of discovery?"

"It was hearsay."

"Yes or no Mrs. Smith."

"No."

"Are you aware that under this same act, you are under obligation to report suspected or witnessed acts of abuse?"

"No, I was not aware."

"What is your understanding of the purpose of the Patient Abuse Hotline?"

"It is a toll free number that can be called to report patient abuse."

"Who should call this hotline number?"

"I thought it was for families, visitors and patients to use."

"If you saw abuse, what do you believe you should do?"

"I would document the incident and notify my supervisor. In nursing we traditionally follow a chain of command."

"Where were you taught to follow a chain of command?"

"In nursing school. In every job I've ever held."

"Did they teach you to follow a chain of command during your orientation here at this nursing home?"

"I don't recall it being part of a formal lesson."

"Do you recall being taught about the patient abuse hotline during your orientation?"

"I recall them discussing the need to report patient abuse. I remember them pointing out the Patient Abuse Posters in the hallways during the tour."

"Do you recall being told during orientation that you must call the patient abuse hotline if you suspected or witnessed any patient abuse?"

"No, I do not recall."

"Have you witnessed or heard of any other cases of patient abuse while under employment of this nursing home?"

"No, I have not."

"Is there anything else you feel we should be aware of at this time?"

"Not that I can think of."

"Thank you Mrs. Smith. You may go. We may have more questions for you at a later time."

I rose to leave then hesitated, "Am I in trouble here?"

The state investigators looked up.

"You failed to report the patient abuse to the hotline, which as a professional nurse you were obligated to do. We'll be in touch."

I decided that this was not the time for pleading or arguing. If I hadn't mentioned what this aide had told me, I wouldn't have been in this mess. I had no idea if Rebecca really saw it happen or not. I had no way of knowing if what Rebecca thought she saw really was a slap. What I now knew was that all that didn't matter. I was supposed to have called the Patient Abuse Hotline myself.

I walked down the hall in a daze. My license to practice nursing was hanging in the balance. I had visions of trying to get employment with a Master's Degree in Nursing without a license. Being in school at the time, I was thinking of the thousands of dollars in debt that I was accruing, potentially in vain.

I waited for the elevator, wallowing in self-pity, absorbed with my own thoughts, staring blankly. Suddenly, words on the poster in front of me jolted me back into consciousness.

"PATIENT ABUSE HOTLINE"

A week too late, I read the fine print.

"Any suspected or witnessed abuse...patients, family, visitors, friends, hospital personnel.. 1-8OO-...Any persons calling in good faith will be free from persecution ..."

Everything the state investigator had said was true, written in black and white. I had walked past this poster hundreds of times before, but never once had actually read it. Now I wish I had. When I got back to the floor, Sara was chatting with one of the day supervisors. They called me over.

"How did it go?" Sara asked.

"They read me my rights. I think I'm going to get a lawyer."

"They read me my rights too. It really scared the s.. out of me. I can't believe this is really happening," Sara said shaking her head.

"The nursing home has lawyers for us," the supervisor explained. "It isn't necessary to get your own. That is what Respondeat Superior is all about."

Respondeat Superior is a legal clause that requires employers to accept responsibility for the actions of its employers, providing house policies are followed.

"This seems to be a gray area," I told her. "I'm not going to take a chance."

Sara joined in, "Yeah. If it came down to the administration or us, I would think the lawyers will remember which side their bread is buttered on."

The supervisor responded, "I'm not going to get my own lawyer for this. The state is always trying scare tactics with nursing homes. I've been here a long time. The administration will stand behind us."

"Did they read you your rights?" I asked her.

"Not yet. I'm scheduled for later."

"Let's see how you feel about it then."

That night when I got home, I called a friend who was a lawyer and he carefully reviewed all the facts of my case. He didn't think it was going to amount to anything more that a scare tactic either, but we made a complete record of the event for filing purposes anyway.

At work over the next few days, the administrative offices were kept busy by the young and eager state sleuths who had begun a full scale investigation of our "in-house investigation" process. Apparently this had been the modus operandi for some time, even after the new Patient Abuse Reporting Law had gone into effect. By the end of the week, it was apparent that Sara and I were the least of the states' concern. One day when I was down by the main offices, I passed where the investigator was working. He looked up and smiled at me when I passed. Seizing the opportunity I asked, nonchalantly, "How's it going?"

"Interesting. Sorry to scare you and your friend so badly the other day."

"Does that mean I'm not in trouble?" I asked.

"We were trying to get the nursing home to understand that we are serious about this Patient Abuse Reporting Act. We used you to set an example to others. The nursing homes have to let us conduct the investigations and determine if it is warranted or not. That is the law."

"I see. Well you sure taught me. If it's any consolation, I've told everybody I know about the need to report abuse via the hotline."

"That's good to hear."

"Thanks for telling me. Sara and I have been really worried that we were going to lose our licenses."

"Between you and me, it's not YOUR license we are after."

"I noticed," looking around at the stacks of papers gathered on a multitude of carts.

Armed with such wonderful news, I danced back up the steps to my floor and shared what I knew with Sara. The next week, the supervisor stopped by, looking worried.

"My husband and I think that maybe I should get my own lawyer. Do you guys think I can trust the one from the nursing home?"

Fear always provides a unique perspective on a situation.

I resigned the nursing home several months later. Partly because I had other job opportunities arise. Partly because I decided that one close call was enough. On my last day, I looked around at the patients lining the halls, knowing that tomorrow, despite my absence, all would appear the same. It had been an interesting diversion on my career path. Working with a creative staff that had been so responsive to the real needs of their geriatric clientele had been a wonderful learning experience.

I stood at the elevator and read the now infamous poster one last time, smiling. As the elevator doors opened for me to leave, Sam the Weatherman looked up.

"25% chance of showers this evening."

"I'm going to miss you Sam. It's been an honor to know you."

We shook hands.

"Why is it that the cute ones always leave?"

I gave him a kiss on his cheek and was gone. Jack the flirt, looking on, would have to eat his heart out.

I filed the lawyer's papers away, wrongly assuming they would never be needed again. About two years later, a subpoena to appear at a hearing on the issue arrived in my mailbox. My lawyer came with me. Once immunity from prosecution was secured, I shared what I knew.

Two years had made my recollections murky and I was thankful for the notes we had made. Even still, the judge and lawyers looked at me as though I was stupid and incompetent when I hesitated to provide minute details or appeared vague with my answers. I can't imagine what it must be like for nurses trying to recall events seven years later.

It turned out that the state was investigating several past cases of unreported abuse that had been discovered following the incident I had reported, not only at my nursing home, but at others as well. The outcome of the hearings was never revealed to me, though admittedly I didn't research it out on my own.

I suspected, however, that the outcome of these investigations laid the groundwork for some legislation passed ten years later mandating continuing education on the Patient and Child Abuse Reporting Act. All professionals licensed by the state, including nurses, doctors, teachers, and others had to learn about the hotline and need to report. While sitting in the classroom, I heard many people complain about having to take this mandatory course. They didn't know how lucky they were to learn their lesson the easy way.

"Like one who seizes a dog by the ears is a passer-by who meddles in a quarrel not his own."

Proverbs 26:17

PART TWO:

NURSING FROM THE SIDELINES

14

Students at the Helm

"Who told you we had a position?" Helen asked me after inviting me to sit in the chair next to her desk.

"I didn't know if you had an opening or not. I just stopped by to see if you had any teaching opportunities I might be qualified to apply for."

"Jean, come in here a minute. I want you to be in on this too."

Helen had beckoned to a woman passing in the hallway. I stood as the woman entered, as I did my pen fell to the floor from my lap. I picked it up and extended my hand to say hello.

"Karen, meet Jean. She is our Level II Team Leader. That is where we teach all of our medical-surgical nursing."

"Nice to meet you," I said as we all found our chairs.

I could feel Jean looking me over. Jean herself was impeccably dressed, her shoes and purse perfectly complimenting her outfit. My attempt to dress smart for the interview paled in comparison.

"Jean, Karen is interested in teaching for us. From her clinical experience, it looks like she is best suited to your level. She has never taught before. Do you think she could handle it?"

"Can I see her resume?"

Helen passed the paper to her.

"Critical care.. looks good to me." Jean looked at me again. "You look so young."

Jean was reading again. "Says here you are a student in a master's program. What track?"

"I'm going for Clinical Specialization in Critical Care Nursing."

"Why not Education?"

"I'm planning to take all the education courses anyway as electives. I thought it would be better if I had the stronger clinical background even if I do decide to teach."

Helen asked Jean, "So what do you think?"

I felt like I should step out. It seemed odd to hear them work towards a decision in my presence.

Jean nodded, "Let's give her a try. She seems bright and she's got a strong clinical background. She can do it. Do you need me anymore?"

Helen waved, "No, go on. I'll need to talk with you later though about something else."

Jean stopped in the doorway, "Nice to meet you."

"You too," I replied.

I was hired.

The course was taught using a team approach with Jean, her new full-time partner Linda and me. It included lectures, an on-campus simulated laboratory experience, and clinical days in the hospital. I was to serve as the Clinical Instructor for two groups of students. As the clinical instructor, I was expected to research in advance so that I would know everything about the patients I had selected for the students and then validate that the students were prepared to care for the patients before our shift began.

I hadn't been nervous about the actual clinical shift portion until Jean and Linda told me stories of things that had gone awry for them over the years. I sounded impossible to be in so many places at the same time. They told me to hope that while I was with one student, the other ones were doing what they were supposed to be doing.

The least glamorous portion of my job was to review and grade a mountain of weekly student care plans. I could still remember how I hated writing these tedious papers as a student. But Linda and Jean pointed out how it would let me "climb into" the student's heads and see whether or not they were making appropriate connections of theory to practice. It was an odd feeling to find out that something I had long thought such a waste of time really did have merit.

Both Jean and Linda, who was an experienced teacher, were wonderful role models and mentors. Jean exuded self-confidence and was an excellent public speaker. Linda was a patient listener and counselor. They were expert test item writers and knew pathophysiology backwards and forwards. They spent precious time coaching me how to pick patients, run conferences and work with the students. They helped me orient to the Medical Center and to establish myself with the staff nurses and key administrators. When my orientation was over, I felt quite ready for this new job as Clinical Instructor.

I was to have eight students the first day. I assigned one patient each to six of the students and had split the medications from the floor between the other two students. The floor was an isolation unit, so although it had only 24 beds, many of the patients were receiving multiple antibiotic intravenous medications.

Jean stopped by around noon to see how I was doing on my first day. It's hard to describe the look on her face when she found me, draped with miniature IV bags pre-filled with antibiotics.

"You decided to give meds today?" she asked, stunned.

"Weren't we supposed too?" I asked, also stunned.

"I'm sorry. We must have forgotten to tell you. I just assumed... No, we don't usually assign medications until the students have oriented themselves to the floor a bit."

"Oh. I wish I had known. It makes sense."

Jean hesitated, and then asked, "Why do you have so many IV's hanging all over you?"

"These are all due at noon."

Kelly, my student medication nurse came up to us at this point. She looked harried.

"I finished 2B, is that the one for 3A?"

"Yes, Kelly. Get the medication kardex and I'll meet you in the room."

"Okay," Kelly said as she took one of the IV's off my shoulder and scurried back down the hallway.

"Do you mind if I ask how many patients you assigned for meds?" Jean ventured.

"I gave Kelly the North side and Bonnie the South."

Jean's eyes grew even wider.

"You assigned the entire floor?"

"How many do you usually assign?"

"About five patients per student."

"Oh."

What had I been thinking? Having just come from a nursing home where one medication nurse medicated 48 patients, 12 had sounded fairly reasonable to me at the time. Plus after my own intimidating experiences as a new graduate, I was determined that any of MY students would get plenty of hands on experience in school so they would be prepared to work as soon as they graduated. What I didn't realize as a new instructor is that I didn't have to accomplish that all in the first day!

Jean began to chuckle, evolving gradually into full blown laughter.

"I'm sorry for laughing. I just can't believe you took the entire floor. How are the med nurses doing?"

"They've been busy to say the least. Basically, I haven't seen anyone else all day. Boy do I feel stupid."

"You should!" Jean had a way of saying whatever she thought and getting away with it. "Why don't you ask the staff nurses to help out? They've had their fun already watching you suffer."

"That's a good idea. Thanks, I will."

Jean was right. The staff was more than willing to reassume the meds for one half of the floor. The two students and I easily finished our half with the added pressure removed. Linda stopped by at the end of the day.

"Jean told me about the medication fiasco. Are you okay?"

"We made it through. My first day would have been a little easier without it."

"So would your students."

"Oh well, at least the students went home feeling like pros with medications after today."

"They might think they are, but it isn't a good experience when it's that stressful. They are likely to take short cuts or learn the wrong way to do things," Linda explained.

"I hadn't thought about it that way."

"Many new clinical instructors think they are doing their students a favor to give them lots of skills right away. It's more important that they understand why they are doing something and how to do it right."

Thanks to the collective wisdoms and constant support from Helen, Jean, and Linda, I made it through those first few semesters of teaching and came away having experienced a better "practicum" than my friends enrolled in the teaching track in school. With my Master's Degree completed and my part-timer dues paid, the door to my dream full-time teaching was finally opened to me, a career step that would span fifteen years and nine hundred students.

"When pride comes, then comes disgrace,
but with humility comes wisdom."

Proverbs 11:2

15

The Calm Before the Storm

As I looked over my class roster with my teaching partner, Shelly, we could only wonder what was in store for this next semester. Teaching Nursing I was a crapshoot. Students meeting general college admission requirements were allowed entry into class and clinical. Sometimes luck was kind and I would have a bright cohesive group of mature students. But it only took one really inept student in the group to make a clinical day in the hospital a horrendous experience. The worst possible thing that could happen in a classroom setting would be to have someone act disruptively or get behind in lecture content. But if someone was disruptive, acted inappropriately, or did not follow strict guidelines when giving actual direct patient care, it could mean potential patient harm. Malpractice. Loss of our RN license for failure to supervise properly. The beginning of the semester, before the hectic clinical rotations began, offered us our first opportunity to identify the weaker students.

Students in our Associate Degree program tended to be a very heterogeneous group. They varied in age from those directly out of high school to an occasional retiree fulfilling a lifelong dream. Many were homemakers looking to supplement their family income. Others were single, working parents, whose daily arrival in class represented a triumph over the odds. A small percentage of the students were male, offering a stabilizing influence over the female hormonal cycles. While most of the students were highly motivated, a few hoped that writing their tuition check would represent their greatest effort.

The first four weeks before clinical were vigorous enough to sort out some of those not so serious students. It was an opportunity to see which students were able to pick up new skills quickly and more importantly, those who didn't. It would also become apparent which students lacked the common sense needed to survive and excel in a field that demanded independent thinking.

"Is the dressing changed?" I asked a student who failed to have any common sense.

"No. The kardex says to apply a 4 by 4 dressing, but we are out of them."

"Did you call the supply room to get more?"

"I didn't know I could."

One hour later I asked again, "Did you get the dressing changed yet?"

"No. The supply room is out of stock of 4 by 4's until tomorrow."

"So now what?" I asked hopefully.

"I was going to change it tomorrow."

"What dressings do we have in stock today that we might be able to use?"

"I didn't think of that."

It was also our responsibility and privilege to establish the mindset of these new nurses. Shelly and I chose teaching methods that prioritized and valued empathy and patient comfort. That was the kind of nurse that we wanted to produce. That was the kind of nurse I would want taking care of me.

Teaching the students to be compassionate with even the simplest of skills was a constant challenge. Since we initially worked with mannequins, it was easy for the students to become extremely focused on the technical aspects of the skill and lose sight of the patient. It wasn't unusual to see anxious students transfer this mannequin neglect to their real patients.

"Hold your leg up Mrs. Green. I'm almost done," the student requested of an 80 pound, 90 year old woman, whose thigh was beginning to quiver with exhaustion.

"Is this always so difficult?" another asked as they fumbled roughly with the patient's tracheostomy tube. The patient's face was turning deep reddish blue as they were caught mid cough, both hands clawed, white knuckled around the side rails. Being cognizant of patient comfort at all times was a habit that needed to be established early.

Our classroom, located in the hospital basement, doubled as a nursing skills laboratory. There were five hospital beds lined up against the walls on one end of the room with curtains that could be used to partition each "hospital unit". Each bed was occupied by life-size mannequin equipped with dozens of pre-drilled holes for practicing everything from catheterization to colostomy care. The genitalia were detachable to allow practice on both gender types. This unfortunately resulted in occasionally misplaced genitalia, especially close to graduation when students felt mischievous or wanted unusual party decorations.

"Karen, we need help here."

The classroom laboratory always felt bumper to bumper during those first few practice sessions. With 27 students and at most three instructors, questions were fielded at a media blitz like pace. Shelly and I were teaching and practicing bed making, hospital style. Shelly was an easygoing gal who had worked with me for several semesters. She was at a bed station surrounded by a group of students awed by a pillow case application trick she learned in her early training, long before I had even graduated from high school. I watched the demonstration one more time, knowing that I still couldn't do it, and then moved to a group calling for help.

"Will we fail if the seams of the sheets are facing towards the patient?" asked an over anxious new student.

"No. It's nice to know that the folded edge could irritate very sensitive skin, but realistically, when you have eight patients, you won't have time to check for seams, let alone make the bed."

This was the student's first lesson on reality. The students gathered around hanging on my every word trusting me to teach them the right way to do things. To them, we were omnipotent. We were everything they wanted to be. It was a wonderful feeling to experience, even though I knew it wasn't realistic and would only last until I got home to my teenagers who would quickly set *that* record straight.

"Do we have to stand at the head of the bed or can we stand at the middle while we put this drawsheet on?" asked another.

"It doesn't make any difference how you do it as long as you remember the principles," I replied.

The student looked disappointed. She wanted a step-by-step

type answer and I knew it. Students preferred a black and white world just like they got in their basic science classes. But a nurse has to apply facts, not recite them.

"Let's review the principles together," I added, pulling out a handout that they had already been given in class that listed the criteria for validating the skills. The students read the sheet.

"But that doesn't tell me where to stand when I'm putting this draw sheet on," said the first student, still holding the sheet in her hand.

"That's because I don't care where you stand," I replied.

"But if I stood too far forward, couldn't the patient fall?" she asked.

"Now you're thinking," I said, smiling. "The principle is to maintain patient safety at all times during a linen change. Can you do that from the foot of the bed? ... Careful now it's a trick question."

The student thought carefully before answering. "If I put the side rail up before I went to the foot or the bed, the patient would be safe."

This gal would make a good nurse; she could think on her own, had common sense and she wasn't afraid to ask questions.

I eventually broke down and showed the students several ways of making the bed properly which followed the principles on the sheet. Seeing the wide range of acceptable performance brought sighs of relief to most students. When a student acted as though choice was the feared enemy, it was a good indicator of a potentially dangerous clinical student.

Following a break, we gathered the students for a lesson on bedpans. After my own personal fiasco years earlier, I had made a point to add formal instruction on this topic to the Fundamentals curriculum.

"I need a volunteer," Shelly began.

"Bill!" chimed several women as they offered a towering burly male student as their sacrificial lamb. Regardless of the actual performance level of any individual student, the male students often dominated the group, either by choice or design.

Bill, obviously flattered, pretended to resist their pushes, and then jumped onto the bed.

"Thanks for volunteering, Bill," Shelly laughed.

Bill gave a sheepish grin as a couple of the other male students made suggestive jeers about how the teacher got him into bed so easy. We let them play out the scene with giggles of varying degrees erupting from the crowd of 27 squished around one bed unit. A subtle, yet important part of the preparatory phase of nursing care is learning to deal with some of the sexuality issues that can make a caregiver uncomfortable. Nurses view and touch total strangers in places generally reserved for intimate relationships. Whether it is the same or cross gender experiences, it takes some getting used to. Humor helps diffuse the students' anxiety as they gradually develop professional demeanors.

"Okay Bill," Shelly began, "you are now a bedridden patient, totally dependent on the nurse."

Bill slumped into the bed eager to play his role well.

"Bill, it's been over an hour since a nurse has been in the room. You really need to use the bedpan. What will you do?"

Bill tried to get the bedpan out of the side cabinet. The class laughed. I quickly put the siderails up, effectively blocking Bill's reach despite his size.

"Imagine how trapped an 87 year old man might feel," I suggested.

Bill flopped back into the bed.

"Use the call light, Bill," one girl suggested.

Bill looked around for the call light. It was on the floor out of reach.

"Unfortunately, this happens more than it should either by accident or by carelessness." In the crowd, heads nodding in agreement. "Let's get Bill on the bedpan."

Shelly demonstrated the technique to the class using the large metal bedpan.

"Ever used one of these before?" she asked Bill.

"No. Do people actually go on this thing?"

"Not easily. Now you know why so many of our patients are constipated. Do you know how it feels when you go away on vacation and you can't go until you get home to your own potty?" The class chuckled. "Well, imagine being stuck in the hospital for a long time."

Bill was still on the metal pan. "Can I get off this thing?"

"Just a minute, I'll be there as soon as I can," my tone mimicked one heard too often on a busy unit. Then aside to Bill, "Just be thankful you have your clothes on. These metal pans get pretty cold in the winter."

"Aren't you supposed to warm them?" someone asked.

"If they are cold put a little warm water in them in the bathroom to warm it up. It's nice to do, especially for the elderly who are really sensitive to the cold. Alright Bill, let's get you off now."

Shelly completed the demonstration of the bedpan removal technique with special emphasis on the prevention of back splash secondary to butt stick per my request. She procured another "volunteer".

"Cindy, you are next. We are going to try a fracture pan on you."

This was a smaller pan designed for patients who could not tolerate the hip flexion required to sit on the standard large pan.

"Eww," Cindy said. "It feels like I'd be sitting in my own pee with this one."

"You are right. So what is really important to remember with this kind?"

"I hope you'd wash my butt when I finished."

"A little toilet paper isn't enough with this one," she replied.

The crowd, "Ewwed."

"Okay, now you all try it. BOTH kinds. I want you to practice putting someone else on and off the bedpan and to sit on each kind yourself, long enough to know what it feels like."

The crowd began to disperse into small groups and the volume of chatter began to rise.

"Also," I said, now in my teacher shouting voice, "when you are on the bedpan, position yourself so that you feel like you could actually go. It will help you understand why your patients make you rearrange them so much!" The students had stopped briefly to hear what I said, and then eagerly went on with their assignment.

"Nurse, I need a bedpan, NOW!" one student whined.

"I'll be back to take you off in a minute," was heard coming from another group of students.

"Wow, this is really uncomfortable," said a thin student.

"Watch out for my incision," one barked.

A heavy student complained, "You don't have it on right, it's cutting into my left thigh."

All in all the students were actually having fun as they teased and prodded each other and assumed various positions on the metal and plastic thrones. They learned firsthand how awkward a bedpan was for the patient. It was their first lesson on compassion.

The next exercise was a lesson on restraining patients. New skills were commonly introduced using a video. The restraint video showed how to properly secure various types of restraints using totally participating actors. To me, this was not real life. After all, docile patients would not need to be restrained. So during the practice of this skill, I decided it would be more fun for the students to try and restrain a totally berserk patient.

The first time I tried this with a class, I played the part of the berserk patient. But the students really needed help to show them what to do for the exercise to work. I would need a volunteer...

"Bill," I approached quietly, "would you be willing to play the role of a berserk patient?"

"When and where?" he responded eagerly.

"Once I warn the students."

"With pleasure!"

I waited until most of the students had finished circulating around the various Restraint Lab stations set up by Shelly before I interrupted the serene learning environment and told them what was about to happen.

"We need to get the patient back to a bed, apply a chest restraint and wrist/hand restraints. The key here is to do this without hurting the patient or getting hurt ourselves."

"Who are we going to restrain?" someone asked, innocently.

"That's your cue, Bill."

Bill was a challenging berserk patient. He happened to be incredibly stronger than he even looked and within a minute had broken loose from two separate groups of six students as well as a group of three men. He charged out the classroom door and was a hundred feet down the hallway before I reached him to call him back.

"Okay Bill. Great job. Come on back. Can we try it again, but this time, no running away?"

His exalted macho status clearly established, he gave the students a break. It took about ten people just to get Bill on the bed. Getting the restraints on required teamwork and planning. Shelly and I guided the students from the sidelines, wondering if they were really trying as hard as they looked. Most were grimacing and several were working up a significant sweat. Eventually I jumped in to relieve a fatigued student who had been assigned to hold down Bill's right arm. Soon I was grimacing and sweating as well. I couldn't help but be thankful that this exercise was not for real. No sooner would we get one arm in the chest restraint, which fit like a backward vest jacket, Bill would break his other arm loose and undo the previous effort. Finally we had all limbs tightly secured and Mike, another large male student laid over Bill's chest to allow for the final application of the chest posey. Bill struggled for a while longer, in vain. The class cheered.

"He was strong," Shelly whispered to me. "I sure wouldn't want to meet him in a dark alley."

"I hope he passes!" I responded.

Bill finally resting quietly asked, "Did I get an A, Karen?"

"Whatever you want, Mister Bill," I teased back.

"Karen, it's not really like that on the floor is it?" asked a wide-eyed recruit, fresh from high school.

"It's certainly not very common, but I saw some pretty wild patient situations in ICU. When guys went into DT's, that is alcohol withdrawal, we'd use leather restraints to hold them down. It was really wild when the doctors would order a Lumbar Puncture on some guy in DT's. It would take six of us to keep them still even with the restraints on. But no, Alice, the truth is somewhere between. Patients are more often confused than combative."

"Thank goodness," Alice replied.

"This was a good exercise though. You can see it wasn't easy to do it without hurting Bill. By the way, Mike probably shouldn't have laid over top of a patient's rib cage like that. Number one, patients can't breathe and number two, it could break something."

"I wondered about that," Mike repli1ed.

"Can I get out yet?" Bill interrupted.
"Only if you promise to be good," Shelly responded.

While the students read about the skills and practiced and studied and practiced again under the watchful eyes of both peers and instructors, they were inevitably absorbed into the technical side of things. We watched to see who, despite the odds, could continue to consider the patient's needs first. Those who did would make the best nurses.

Fortunately for us all, there are always a few.

"Let us consider how we may spur one another on toward love and good deeds."

Hebrews 10:24

16

Testing... 1,2,3

Before the students were even allowed to touch a real patient, they were formally validated on their ability to perform several basic skills; handwashing hospital style, bedmaking and bedbaths. Complicated skills were taught once this rite of passage was completed.

Most of the students walked in the classroom expecting these first skills to be a cakewalk. After all, everyone did these daily chores by rote at home. But in the classroom they were told they had to wash their hands a specific length of time, rinse in a specific direction, clean to a specified distance above the wrist, not turn off the water faucets until after drying their hands and then only by using a towel. The students were also forced to learn new ways to make beds and bathe. The "more mature", i.e. older students expected to be able to apply years of prior experience but instead found themselves faced with the difficult task of modifying decades of habit.

Each validation exam was an unavoidable stressful experience in the life of a nursing student. The students did not receive a grade, but instead were expected to pass all criteria successfully. One breach of a principle meant failure and required revalidation. Just knowing that you were being watched could turn even the most skilled nurses into jelly. No matter how light a mood I would try to provide to relax the students, it was often to no avail.

Some students shook so uncontrollably, I had to help steady their hands. Some would interject, "I'm so nervous," after every phrase. Sometimes the nervousness was not apparent unless the student was asked a question, only to discover that thinking or speaking outside safe boundaries of their prepared scripts was impossible for them. Occasionally a student walked in, announced they couldn't do it and would leave. Many reported stress responses such as diarrhea, migraines, insomnia, and stomach problems or even broke out in visible hives.

In preparation for a long morning of testing, I positioned a desk chair unit between two bed set-ups. I drew the curtains on either side of the beds for privacy. The curtain in between the beds was pulled just far enough for me to view two students simultaneously. The linens were stacked high on tables behind me, along with extra soap, lotions and mouth care necessities. The first two students, Brittany and Cindy, were the eager beaver type. They had both been practicing together in the practice lab for endless hours the week prior to the validation. They performed the skills perfectly, often quoting the videos. Although the students were allowed 45 minutes to complete this skill, they both completed the skills test in record times, 31 and 32 minutes respectfully.

I gestured to Shelly a thumbs up and mouthed, "Excellent". Shelly shook her head and rolled her eyes upward in response, indicating that she hadn't been so lucky on her first go round.

Liz started off the second round of students. Her lack of confidence contrasted sharply with the performance of Brittany and Cindy. She bumbled around changing her mind frequently as to what she would do next, catching herself before she made errors in technique. By the time Liz was finished giving her mannequin the bedbath, she had perspiration rolling down her forehead. I couldn't resist giving her an extra dry washcloth.

"Did I miss something?" Liz asked anxiously.

"No, your bath was fine, Liz. That's for your forehead."

"Oh," she said, unaware that a big drip had just fallen from her onto her mannequin's face.

I wondered whether perspiring onto a patient breached the validation criteria, but decided quickly that to even mention it even in jest would devastate her.

"Make sure you carry a tissue for your brow when you give a bath Liz. Sometimes it gets real hot behind the curtains."

"I usually do," she replied. "It was just that I was so nervous today, I forgot to. I sweat so easily."

"You are doing fine. Let me see you make the bed."

Liz took a deep breath and began preparations for making the bed, occupied by the mannequin. I turned my attention to Bill, who had begun his validation shortly after Liz, and was busy washing the mannequin in the adjacent bed. He was slopping water from a very drippy washcloth across the mannequin's leg on the way to the chest. I made a note on my sheet. I wondered what else I had missed while talking with Liz. Bill finished washing the feet then stopped abruptly.

"Oh, I would have put a towel underneath the feet if this had been a real patient."

"Bill, during validation, this IS a real patient."

Bill scrambled and put a towel under the feet. If that had been his only error, I would not have failed him, since he remembered it on his own. But the list on my scratch pad continued to grow. Bill began to clean the mannequin's perineal area, never stopping to change the water or the washcloth after he'd washed the feet. Textbooks will cite the theory of always cleaning from the cleanest area to the dirtiest. Most would call it common sense. Patients would not want what was on the bottom of their feet wiped on their perineal area. Bill was going to need careful watching in the clinical area... and more practice in the lab.

"Bill, you've made several mistakes already. You will need to repeat this part of the validation. Why don't you just go on and make the bed."

"What do you mean, several mistakes?"

I listed off each breach of principle that I had observed.

"You didn't offer the patient a bedpan prior to starting the bath."

"I did when you were talking with Liz, you didn't see me."

"Okay then," giving him the benefit of much doubt, "you left the side rail down when you went to get your sheets off the chair. That's number six, "Maintain patient safety at all times."

"I was only a few feet away. I could get back if the patient started to fall." Bill demonstrated his speed.

"First, if the chair was further away, like in most patient rooms, you might not be able to get back so quick. Second, it's a bad habit to go anywhere without pushing up the bedrail. Lastly, that's not what you were taught."

Bill's neck and face deepened to a reddish hue as he took on a defiant mask, commonly seen in adolescents.

"Anything else?" he sneered.

"You didn't prepare your washcloth properly to maintain the comfort of the patient."

"My hand is too big to make the mitt Shelly taught us."

"I didn't say you needed to make a mitt. You slopped water across the sheets and the patient's exposed body areas because the washcloth was too wet."

"I'm going to change the sheets anyway."

"In the meantime, you didn't maintain the comfort of the patient. That was criteria number seven."

Bill sighed deeply, still defiant.

"Lastly, you washed the perineal area with the foot water. That was criteria number five, change water when dirty."

"I would have changed the water after the feet," Bill countered. "I assumed you knew that."

"Bill, you need to either say that you would change the water or actually do it."

"I didn't think we were allowed to."

"I don't know where you got that idea. Your classmates all seemed to understand that."

"Well, Shelly told us we didn't have to."

Team teaching can be a real advantage to quick thinking manipulative students. Unfortunately for him, Shelly and I communicated closely and were wise to such deceptive methodology.

"Excuse me for a second."

I motioned to Shelly who was sitting in her own two-bed cubicle. Joining us, I asked her to verify Bill's statement, which I suspected was false. Bill took the offensive.

"Shelly, didn't you tell us in lab that we would not need to actually change the water?"

Shelly, forced to agree with this added, "Yes, but you were also told you needed to tell us when you would change the water."

"On the video they did it differently then you showed us in class. I followed the video."

"The sequence for the bath is clear on your validation preparation sheet."

"I didn't use that, I went by the video," Bill insisted.

Danielle, a well-prepared student who was being tested by

Shelly on the other side of the curtain, poked her head around.

"The video was a little different, but they still changed the water after the feet."

Hardworking students were often resentful of those who flaunted their laziness and would gleefully contribute to their demise.

Bill looked around sharply at her. "Thanks a lot." He raised his voice. "These validations are so unreal. I've taken care of real patients before. This pretending doesn't reflect what I'd really do. This is ridiculous. Are you telling me that I have to do this whole thing again?"

In Bill's defensive posture, he had missed the whole point of the validation exercise.

"Thanks Shelly," I said, dismissing her. "Bill, sit down. Let's just talk a second."

Bill came closer but refused to sit and give up his obvious height advantage. I spoke in a low, calm voice, hoping to portray a firm, yet friendly tone.

"We do not do validations to get you upset or to make you feel attacked. We do this so that YOU can know that what you are doing with patients is correct. Also, when we go to the floors next week, and you do a bath on a real patient, I need to know that you can work safely on your own."

"I'll be fine with real patients."

"I'm sure you will be, but today you were not able to demonstrate to me that you knew how to give a hygienically sound, safe, and comfortable bath. So.. Let's review some things so there is no further confusion of what you are expected to do for us."

"Imagine you are an elderly patient who became incontinent of urine on the way to the bathroom, stepping inadvertently in puddles of urine. When the nurse washes you, when would you like your water changed?"

"After the feet."

"When else?"

"I don't know."

The more I quizzed him, the more I realized how little preparation he had done. His initial fight had been to save face and create a distraction from the truth. He had tried to wing it, and he was caught.

"Leg, foot, leg, foot?" Shelly peeked around the curtain again.

"Leg, leg, foot, foot, change," I replied. "If you did leg, foot, leg, foot, the water would be dirty for the second leg."

"Mary said we said leg, foot, leg, foot. I thought it was leg, leg, foot, foot, but I couldn't remember anymore. I need some coffee," Shelly said pretending to look dazed.

Turning back to Bill I said, "Let's see you make the bed."

I looked over and watched Liz as she struggled to tuck the sheets under her mannequin. The plastic mannequin had insufficient weight to keep the new sheet pinned under it. Every time she positioned the sheets under the upper torso, the lower torso sheets would loosen. Liz stopped to mop her drippy brow in a panic. This scene had probably been going on the entire time I had been distracted with Bill.

"A real patient will be heavy enough to hold the sheet for you," I explained, attempting to diffuse her anxiety.

"I practiced with the other mannequins. They were heavier."

"Here, let me help."

I got up and added some weight to the mannequin by leaning on it. Her sheets were on within minutes, much to Liz's relief. I checked my watch. Fifty minutes had passed. Although she was beyond the time limit, I let it slide on account of the prolonged sheet battle she had fought.

"Good job Liz, you are all set."

"I passed?"

"Yes, you passed."

"Really?"

"Really."

"Oh thank you, thank you, thank you," she said clapping her hands, face beaming. "I've been making my kids and husband in their beds all weekend! They'll be so relieved to know they can stop!"

She started out of the testing room then turned and came back. She whispered in my ear, "Don't worry, I promise I'll always carry a dry washcloth with me."

"Good."

I peeked over at Bill before calling my next student. He was making the bed quickly and correctly. He raised and lowered the side rails several times, looking at me to make sure that I noticed his careful attention to patient safety. I went in the hall to get Caitlin. Caitlin jumped when she heard her name.

"Your turn."

I had already identified Caitlin as one of the weaker students. Caitlin had shadowed several other stronger students throughout the practice sessions and avoided doing the skills herself, unless asked. She didn't ask any questions, perhaps because she already felt so overwhelmed, she wouldn't know where to start or what to ask.

"Where do I go?" she asked timidly.

"You'll wash the patient in this bed," I said pointing. "Then change the sheets."

"Can I get my linens first?"

"That would probably make it easier," trying not to sound too sarcastic.

Bill had finished his bed and now stood waiting for me, making no attempt to hide his obvious disgust with the situation. I walked to the bed and checked his corners then pulled a quarter out of my pocket.

"Do you think it will bounce?" I teased, tossing the coin on the bed. The coin landed face up.

"Heads, you pass this part. Great bed, Bill. I can tell you've done this before."

Bill accepted the praise more willingly than the prior corrections. I handed him a slip that listed his errors and the time for his revalidation appointment. These retests were scheduled purposely on a non-class day. After years of teaching, I had resorted to the same tactics I had once despised and questioned of my earlier role models. There was no denying that when the retest time was inconvenient, the preparation for the first test increased dramatically.

Bill looked at the slip. "I don't have class that day. Can't I do it before or after class on Wednesday? I might have to work."

"It's scheduled during a time you were told to keep open. I'll see you on Tuesday."

Had he pushed I probably would have backed off. We tried to work around work schedules whenever we could, but Bill had pushed me too far already today. Unless I wanted to be manipulated the entire semester, I knew from experience to stand firm.

Bill grabbed his books and huffed out. He could be heard sharing some expletives with the students in the hallway, but they dismissed him quickly. After two weeks of intense coursework and lab practice, his fellow students had already figured him out and lacked sympathy for his disappointments.

Caitlin was still selecting linens when I came back in with Dale, an LPN.

"Let's get this over with so I can get to work," Dale said to me. "Which bed do I do?"

Her flippant attitude was not uncommon for students with many years of nursing experience who felt forced to return to school. Although the LPN background often made the mandatory clinical experiences much easier for these returning students, the RN program covered the content material at a much greater depth. There were higher expectations for applying theory to clinical practice as well as independent decision making. I never had an LPN tell me they had wasted their time or hadn't learned a great deal in any RN nursing course.

My approach to the LPN students during the first few weeks of the program was to help them get comfortable resuming the learner role and to let them know that their prior knowledge was valuable. I often asked them if they would be willing to assist the "less experienced students". I solicited their feedback on current practice where they worked as points of comparison or validation to what we were teaching. Occasionally an LPN had a unique way of doing a skill that was an improvement to what we were teaching. I would let the LPN share this or present it myself as an acceptable alternative, giving the student appropriate credit.

Once the LPN began to feel more like a colleague, they would relax long enough to discover what I already knew. That their LPN programs had only scratched the surface of knowledge and two more years of intensive study would only put a dent into all that could be learned about assessment, pathophysiology, disease management, and the art and science of nursing. Learning in nursing is a life-long process.

Dale's chip on the shoulder attitude was based on a tremendous self-confidence that would ultimately serve her well.

I smiled, knowing she could do this skill with her eyes closed, but the time would come when she would be on par with the others.

"I don't think it will take that long Dale. Work on the bed on the left."

Dale had entire validation completed before Caitlin finished the upper half of her bath. It had taken Caitlin ten minutes just to maneuver the bath blanket into place and to get the gown off.

Linda entered the testing area vacated by Dale. Linda was classy by anyone's standards. She was in her forties, owned a successful business, but wanted to pursue her childhood dream to be a nurse. She was a smart looking gal and was always tastefully dressed. She knew how to handle herself around others, displaying a well-timed sense of humor. She worked hard for her grades and constantly sought out and accepted critique.

"Do you mind if I talk to the mannequin while I work? It helps me relax," she asked.

"Anything that works is fine with me."

"Hello Mrs. Jones," Linda began using a comforting tone. "My name is Linda and I'm here to assist you with your bath this morning. I heard you had a tough night. Uhh huh. Ohh. Is the pain any better? Uhh huh. Yes. I'll mention it to the medication nurse while I get your linens. Is there anything else I can get for you?" She paused, as if listening to a reply. "Sure, I'll bring an extra box of tissues. Do you need a garbage bag too?"

Linda's patient focused one-way patter was unusually entertaining. She continued this way through her mouth care and the upper body bath in a manner that would have put even the most timid patient at ease. This student was the kind of nurse I would want to take care of me.

"Now, Mrs. Jones, it's time to clean your private area. Can you do it or would you like me to help? " She nodded. "You'd like me to help. Sure, that's what we are here for."

Linda pulled back the blanket exposing the genitalia.

"Oh me! Oh my Mrs. Jones!" Linda exclaimed in a shocked voice as she looked down at the mannequin's penis. Then in a quick recovery, returning to the same calm patter, she continued, "Now when exactly is the sex change operation scheduled for? Oh great. You must be eager to be done with this."

I lost it at that point. Passive observation was not my forte anyway. Linda, seeing her instructor erupt with laughter, joined in as she finished drying the eternally erect penis, covered it up, patted it and then claimed, "All clean!"

Caitlin in the meantime had reached the end of her 45-minute time limit but was not even close to finishing the bath. I conferred with Shelly and we decided to let her finish for practice since we were ahead of schedule, but that she would not pass.

Linda, having recovered from her shock moved on with style and grace. She began changing the sheets while I took a few moments to show Caitlin some things. When I returned to my post, Linda, who apparently had difficulty positioning the mannequin to stay on it's side, had draped an arm and a leg over the side rails, it's face pressed down into the pillow.

"I know it looks hideous Karen, but the mannequin just won't stay over."

"As long as I don't see you do that with a real patient, I'll let it slide," I replied.

Just then I heard a loud bang come from the other side of the room. I ran over to find a mannequin body lying on the floor, legs still in the bed. The student, horrified, hand on her mouth, stared on. She probably thought that her career as a nurse was ended.

"I killed the mannequin!" she exclaimed. "It fell apart when I gave him a bath and when I turned him over to put on the sheets, his arm flipped over the rail and took the body with him."

Shelly, having arrived behind me, began to chuckle.

"Looks like this guy needs an order for a chest restraint," Shelly said.

"Do we have a criteria that says the nurse should not remove patient legs during a bath without a signed consent?" I asked.

Our assistant instructor offered, "It really wasn't her fault. The mannequin disintegrated in front of her. She had the side rail up and was doing everything correctly."

I walked to the student and patted her back. "It's okay, really. Trust me, you'll laugh about this someday too."

I had the rest of my students validated, the entire lab cleaned up, and had even washed the dingy blackboards and the filthy window sills before Caitlin finished her bath and bed in a record one hour and forty-five minutes.

"You did everything correctly, Caitlin," I counseled. "We just need to pick up the speed a little."

"When can I retake the validation?"

"It's on this slip here. Caitlin please promise me that you will make at least ten beds for practice before you come back on Tuesday."

"I will. Thank you for letting me stay today."

"No problem."

Caitlin gathered all of her stuff. I turned off the classroom lights and waited in the doorway for her. I sighed, thinking that this girl was hopelessly slow. I wondered how she ever thought she would survive in a fast paced stress filled career such as nursing. Watching her pile up a stack of textbooks with her frail frame, it seemed that a librarian career would be more fitting. But it wasn't for me to decide. Her choice had been made. It was up to me to give her a fair shot at her goal.

As we walked down the dreary corridor with a ceiling of exposed plumbing and electrical lines, she asked me quietly, "Do you think I've got a chance of making it? The other students seem to catch on so much quicker than I do."

"Ohh," wondering if she'd just read my mind, "it just takes some people longer than others. Give yourself a chance to get the hang of it. Someday you'll be taking care of six to eight patients on a unit and not even bat an eye. You just need practice. You'll get faster, you'll see."

"Do you really think so?"

"I know so. Every time you do it, you'll get a little faster, then a little faster. So what if you have to do something ten times in practice when someone else can do it in two. Who cares? The important thing is that you do it in the end. It's even more important that you know what you are doing and why it's being done.

Caitlin nodded, wheels turning. "I understand the readings. I did well on the quizzes so far too. That part of it I can handle."

"So that's where you start from. Let that be your source of confidence."

We climbed the steps to the main floor of the school. Streams of daylight signaled that we had reached the exit door of the school. Caitlin opened the door bringing in a flood of crisp autumn air.

"Hey," I said, "I'm pulling for you. Now don't YOU give up on yourself."

"Okay, I won't. Thanks Karen," she nodded.

"See ya Tuesday Caitlin."

I passed Shelly's office on my way back to my own.

Seeing me pass, she sighed loudly. "I'm glad that's over with! That was painful. What took you so long?"

I pushed my door open with my foot, dumped my notebook and pens on my desk then came back to her office, a mirror reflection of my own. Our offices were converted dormitory rooms that were built more as sleeping quarters than living spaces with windows overlooking the pharmacy roof laden with an assortment of pipe vents.

"Caitlin just finished her bed."

Shelly looked at her watch.

"Oh my gosh. Who's got her first in clinical?" she asked standing up to check the list posted on her bulletin board. "Phew! You've got her."

"Thanks a lot."

I took the paper down and studied the lists of clinical groups I had made weeks ago. Now that I was able to attach faces and in some cases, abilities to the names, it was like reading it for the first time.

"You've got Bill," Shelly said.

"Did you hear him today?" I asked.

"I couldn't get over what a hard time he gave you. Some students are really bold. I never would have spoken to a teacher like that," Shelly replied.

I read on.

"Thank goodness, I've got Linda. She seems like she is going to be great."

I shared the story about the gender confusion and we had a good stress-relieving laugh.

"What's Amy like?" I asked. "I haven't worked with her much.

"She's very bright and capable, but there's something about her I don't trust." Shelly squinched her brow. "I can't put my finger on it."

"Your instincts are generally good. I'll stay on my toes. Brittany did a great job this morning."

"Some of them look so young don't they?" Shelly observed.

I continued to read down my list. "I know Dale. She's good but she has an attitude."

"Isn't she one of the LPN students?"

"Yeah."

"Danielle's an LPN too, isn't she. Didn't you have her today?"

"Yes," Shelly replied, "and she doesn't have an attitude. She'll be one of your strongest I'll bet. Last week she was very helpful with the others."

"I'm glad to hear that," reading on. "Russell.. do you think "Doc" really knows anything or is he just hot air?"

Shelly shrugged her shoulders. "The adjunct had him today and I really haven't worked with him much." She checked the grade sheet. "He passed with no problems and he has hundreds on the first two quizzes."

"Loretta Limpkin. She seemed nice, very attentive, asked a zillion questions."

"She's the only one who got the sheet seam on right today," Shelly offered. "I remember interviewing her to come here. This is her fourth college program in five years. She started out in vet school then went to beauty school. I can't remember the rest."

"So if this doesn't work out, she could groom sick dogs?"

"There you go."

"Rice, which one was she?"

"She's the flamboyant one with hot pants and heavy make-up. How did you miss her?" Shelly asked.

"I didn't miss her, but I keep blocking on her name. I keep wanting to call her Dana for some reason."

"Dana is the one with the straight black hair that sits in the back and sleeps."

"I'll get them straight eventually."

"Rice is the one who goes "EW, do we really do that?" at least once an hour."

"Do you think she knows what she got herself into?"

"I don't know. Wonder what she wrote on her philosophy paper."

I went next door to my office and came back with a stack of

papers. Students were required to write a short composition to reflect on their personal philosophy of nursing within the first week of the program. The less mature students generally lifted the school philosophy from the student handbook to turn in one that they thought would meet the faculty approval. More mature students often wrote very revealing introspective compositions. Rice's philosophy mirrored the schools but her comments were telling.

"I was laid off from my computer job and my friends suggested I try nursing since it pays well and has good job security," I read.

"There's a lot more to nursing than money." Shelly's face had quickly turned red. "These people don't have a clue. I know I'm old school, but it really makes me angry when I hear that. There's just not the same level of dedication that we had to have in order to get into nursing years ago. I think it shows at the bedside."

"Hold on, hold on. There's more," I told her. "Nursing is an exciting career that allows you to help people."

Shelly barely let me finish.

"Isn't that sweet," Shelly responded in a mocking tone. "I give her two months."

"You're funny!"

Shelly, still heated, shaking her head, replied, "No I mean it."

"I know you do. That why I love working with you. And by the way, I agree with you."

Any two faculty can be teamed up to share course responsibilities, but only a few are lucky enough to have really wonderful partnerships. Shelly and I, despite the difference in our ages, backgrounds, work patterns and methodologies, shared the same philosophies towards education and educating, nursing, and life. It made blowing off steam easy and fun, especially since your opinions were usually reaffirmed, not refuted. It also provided a comfortable mutual base of support for dealing with the myriad of student problems and issues that arose on a regular basis.

Our informal session continued long enough to review Shelly's clinical student group as we had done with mine. By the time we had finished, our feet had managed to sneak up on the desk, striking a lazy, carefree pose for a casual observer. But much was actually accomplished in these sharing sessions that allowed us to be properly prepared for a student clinically. The information gleaned would guide our decisions as to which patients to choose and which students to watch like hawks to insure patient safety.

Working with nine brand new freshman students was never easy. Initially, the odds for disaster were great. These sessions only served to push the odds a little towards our favor. The next week, clinical in the real world, away from the surreal world of laminated patients, would begin.

"A wise man's heart guides his mouth,
and his lips promote instruction."

Proverbs 16:23

17

The Other Side of Fright

I arrived at the hospital as usual, around 6:3O a.m. My students weren't due to arrive until 7:3O. This gave me plenty of time to review any changes in patient status that might have occurred in the 16 hours since I last read their charts. Now, a seasoned instructor, I worked quickly, easing clipboards out from under the protective arms of the night staff, hoping to catch a glimpse of essential data before the day staff claimed the data piles for their own private viewing. If I missed getting a Kardex sheet now, I would not get to see it until at least 8 or 8:30.

I was done with my quick review by 6:45 as the day staff began entering the station. They checked their assignment then whisked the clipboards off to listen to the reports recorded on tape by the night staff.

"The students are back, finally!" one staff nurse remarked as she saw me.

"Just baths and beds today," I said with an apologetic tone.

"Oh, we'll take whatever help we can get. I love having the students around."

Not all the staff felt that way, but enough did on this floor to make it a great learning experience for the students. I made rounds on the floor, leaving post-it notes marked "Freshman Student Nurse" on the patient clipboard boxes outside the rooms in the hall. I did this to help me remember which rooms the nine students were assigned to for the day. The patients were spread across two long hallways that formed an "L" with the nurses' station and utility rooms located in the center. Without the post-it, I sometimes lost track of where they were, especially when things got hectic.

The post-it notes also helped remind the staff to stay clear of a particular patient, especially the nurse's aides who opted out of listening to report in lieu of getting a head start on their work. There was nothing more devastating to a new student than to walk in with a head full of plans and find the patient already bathed and dressed. Students could be reassigned, but few functioned at their personal best with changed circumstances.

By 7:00 a.m., my notes were in place and my prep work was completed. While I waited for the students to arrive, I roved around the various rooms where groups of three or four nurses and aides were clumped to prepare for their teams assignment. I paused any time I heard the name of one of our patients, catching bits and pieces of the report being given. My own research often had given me more information than what was passed verbally in the morning and it was not unusual for me to pass information I had read back to the staff to explain some test or restriction being imposed. My visibility to the staff was probably more important than the actual information I gathered. It was vital that my relationship with staff members be strong in order for me to be an effective clinical instructor.

"Who you got today, Karen?" one RN asked.

"2A, 3A, 4B." I knew that Jackie had Team III, a group of about eight patients.

"Oh good. Watch the guy in 4B. He swings."

"Great. Just what my student needs the first day."

Another nurse spoke up, "He was fine for me yesterday. He's on Mellaril now." Mellaril was a strong tranquilizer.

"I didn't see that," said the RN.

"Phew," I replied. "The gal that has him is afraid of her own shadow."

"You'll whip her into shape in no time."

"I hope so."

Another LPN across the room called, "Karen, how come we didn't get any students today? We have a ton of IV's."

"Sorry about that Sue. Luck of the draw. We needed plain old baths today. Save the fancy stuff for later!"

I checked my watch. It was already 7:30 and not a single student had arrived. Strange, I thought. This group had been very punctual until now.

The secretary of the unit beckoned from the nurses' station,

"Karen, call for you."

Reaching out over the desk I caught the phone as the secretary dashed away. The school secretary was on the line.

"Karen, I've got a nervous group of students here in the school with me. What do you want me to do with them?"

"Tell them that their patients are up here with me, waiting for them."

I heard her pass the message with her own added, "Get going, you'll be fine." She paused as she waited for them to be gone from earshot. "You've got some winners there Karen. Have a good day. They are on their way!"

I walked back into the report room, "Go easy on my students' today guys. They were too afraid to even come to the floor!" As I explained the reason for their late arrival, several chuckled and reminisced of their first days as students.

"Don't worry, we'll go easy on them," Jackie said.

"Oh and by the way, if you see anything, like side rails down, patients half out of bed, you know, first day stuff, don't hesitate to jump in!"

"No problem!" They responded.

It was nice to know that there were several other sets of eyes watching on that first day. I remembered working with instructors who were offended if staff interacted with their students in any way. I don't know how they did it alone.

The students, a group of nine clones with freshly starched uniforms, white shiny shoes, arms loaded with books and dazed looks reflecting a sleepless night wrought with anxiety, rounded the bend.

"Glad you could make it," I said checking my watch. "We'll meet in there," pointing to the only vacant waiting room. Six students sat on the available chairs, the rest stood uncomfortably against the wall. As I walked past, Russell stood to offer me his chair. He was a tall, nice looking man in his mid thirties with an air of experience. His shirt pockets bulged with more equipment than the typical resident physician.

"No thanks," I said, brushing past him as I walked to the ventilator/seat lining the window. "This is fine for me." I motioned to the others, still standing. "Come over and join me, I promise I won't bite."

The students gathered their book bags from the floor and sheepishly sat down on the window ledge, the seats furthest away from me filling first.

"Well good morning! Welcome to clinical. I will say this is the first time I thought my entire group wasn't going to show."

Linda, with her hair swept back neatly in a classic bun, spoke up for the entire group and explained. "We've been downstairs in the school since 7:00. We didn't know we were allowed to come up here by ourselves. We must look pretty stupid."

"First day jitters, that's all. Just think, four hours from now, it will be over with and you won't have to worry about baths or beds anymore."

Rice quietly added, "Yeah, we'll just have to worry about a hundred other things."

I pretended not to hear her.

"Let's get started."

Papers began to rustle.

"Were you able to find all the patient information yesterday?"

Loretta, looking forlorn said, "I didn't understand a lot of what I read, or wrote down for that matter."

Several other students nodded their heads in agreement.

"That's okay. I didn't expect you to the first time. The handwriting isn't easy to decipher is it?"

Again the group nodded.

"Remember, you are learning an entirely new language this semester in addition to everything else. Don't worry, it will come gradually. Your research will give you a chance to get familiar with charts and to learn to speak medspeak."

"I thought it was just me," Linda said.

"Nope. Everybody starts out that way. Do you all have your assignment worksheets?"

I looked around and each student held up a heavily penned in four page worksheet.

"Okay then. I've seen you've done your preparation. I'll look at each of your sheets later. Next week that research will be the focus of our morning conference, but I'll bet that isn't what is on your mind this morning," I said looking around the room. "I think it would be better if we take the next thirty minutes," checking my watch, "make that 22 minutes, to address your concerns this morning. So.. questions? Concerns?"

"I'm really afraid I'm going to hurt somebody." Loretta had spoken first.

"Me too," others echoed.

"Fair enough, what's the worst thing that could happen?"

"They could die," Linda said. Others laughed nervously.

"Alright. We are in a hospital. People do die in hospitals. We are on a hospice floor. People often come here to die. It IS a possibility. The question is not could they die, but what should we do if they die, that is stop breathing."

I looked around the room. The students were leaning forward in their seats, their faces wrought with anxiety. There was no doubt that I held their steadfast attention.

"The first question you need answered before you even enter your patient's room is, is my patient a code or a no code? If they are a hospice patient or a no code and they stop breathing, walk out in the hall and find me or another nurse."

"What if they aren't a no-code," Russell asked. "Do we start CPR? Isn't that why we had to be certified before we came here?"

"Yes and no. If a patient stops breathing, your primary responsibility is to initiate the code alarm. I recommend that you get help. That doesn't mean coming and finding me. It doesn't mean wandering the halls looking for a nurse. It means calling out loudly, HELP in room number whatever. Throw a tray if you need too, that always brings people running."

Russell asked, "Aren't we supposed to pick up the phone and dial the emergency number?"

"What is the number Russell?"

"33."

"Good. How many of you remembered that?"

A few hands went up.

"In a panic, and believe me, having your patient stop breathing will make you panic, the average student nurse would forget her own name."

"Not Russell," Linda added.

"Do we start CPR then?" Russell asked eagerly.

"You bet! You can help position the patient and get the CPR board under them, but once the room fills, get out of the way when asked. Let the experienced nurses take over. So," pausing to look around at the widened eyes of my students, "now you know how to handle the absolute worst thing that can happen today."

Brittany, one of the youngest in the group and obviously very concerned asked, "Has it ever happened to your students before?"

"Not very often, once every couple of semesters maybe. With most patients, there is adequate warning that something is not right. You are not alone on this unit and very little will be expected from you at his point."

The students began to ask a myriad of much more reasonable questions, like whether that could actually talk to the staff nurses or were they allowed to answer call lights of other patients. Practical stuff. The students actually began to relax a little as they each had a chance to ask their real questions in a non-threatening environment. As the pace of the questions slowed, I checked my watch again.

"Follow me," I said leaving the room, hearing a flutter of activity behind me. I led my flock to an empty private room. "Squish in," I directed as all nine managed to fit into a room that was barely large enough to hold the bed and a chair with the door opened into it. "This is the call bell. This is how you turn it off. Take turns. Everybody try it."

With the light intermittently flickering on and off with each students practice, Jackie, the floor nurse, poked her head in the door, her hands filled with medications.

"Need help in here?"

"Sorry Jackie, we're just practicing. We'll be done in a minute."

"Glad to have you here," Jackie said to the students with a smile.

"Good morning," the group said in almost perfect unison.

Jackie laughed. "Well done," she said before taking off down the hall.

I completed the demonstration with a review of the bathroom call light and the bed controls.

Russell stood back, "I know how to work these beds already."

Dale looked bored. She whispered something to Russell then sounding impatient said, "Shelly made us practice the bed controls in lab."

Caitlin looked up, "Some of us aren't experts yet."

I interrupted, blocking the next shot. "Anyone who feels ready to start, head on out. I'll be around to check on you. Try to find me for your questions if you can, so that we don't drive the staff nuts."

Dale, Russell, Danielle and Amy were out the door before I finished talking. Loretta lagged behind for a few more questions then left. Caitlin was still playing with the bathroom call light, Linda patiently showing her once again. Caitlin's stick like frame contrasted sharply with Linda's mature curves. Caitlin's straight mousey brown hair was cut short with little attention to style. Her plain face was noticeably devoid of any make-up.

Rice asked, "My patient is on complete bedrest. What if he needs to go to the bathroom? Can I get him up?"

"Complete bedrest means no getting up. Your patient will have to use a bedpan."

"Oh gross, really?" Rice's face had scrunched. "I'll put him on, but I can't get him off."

Linda had joined us. "At least yours uses the bedpan, my patient is incontinent."

"That's disgusting," Rice responded.

"Yesterday he had just had diarrhea all over the place when I went in to say hello."

"Who has to clean something like that up?" Rice asked.

"The nurses were doing it yesterday," Linda answered.

"Do we students have to do that?"

"Yes, Rice. That's part of nursing."

Rice didn't need to respond verbally. Her non-verbals said it all. She had used only one layer of make-up today, but with her skin tight uniform, she still stood out from the others. Linda left the room chuckling at Rice's response.

Caitlin asked me, "Should I go to my patient's room yet?"

"How about if I go with you?" I responded.

Caitlin looked relieved, "Would you?"

Brittany, still hanging around the group asked, "Me too?"

"Sure, come on. How about you Rice?"

Rice half nodded and followed along. I got to Caitlin's room and entered. Caitlin stood frozen at the door. She was a fragile kind of person and I couldn't help wanting to protect her. I went back, took her by the arm gently and walked her to the bed by the window.

"Good morning, Mr. Peters. You've met Caitlin, your student nurse for today?"

Students had to say hello to their patients the night before as part of clinical preparation.

"I'm Karen, Caitlin's instructor."

Mr. Peters looked at both of us, making a slight grunt of a response before closing his eyes again. I turned to Caitlin.

"Let's review what we have here." I handled each piece of bedside equipment, reviewing its use and necessary nursing care. I pointed out the bed controls and alarms that we had just practiced with. "Let me see your assignment worksheet."

I quickly read through her clinical preparation sheet. "This looks good Caitlin. You know why Mr.Peters is here and your priorities look great. Stick with your plan and you'll do fine."

Caitlin remained frozen at the edge of the bed. I reached into the bedside stand and took out the washbasin and put it into her hands. "Why don't you start by washing him up. Someone has already brought linens in here for you."

Caitlin took the basin and started for the bathroom. Inertia gone, she would be fine. I returned to the hallway and put my arm around Brittany's shoulder.

"Next? Let's go."

Brittany's patient was a middle-aged woman with rapidly diminishing physical abilities as a result of a brain tumor. She had only a few strands of blondish hair on her head, a paisley turban lay crumpled on the bedstand behind some wilting flowers. She was alert but a little cranky this morning.

"Good morning, Mrs. Emerson."

"Who are you?" she barked.

I introduced myself and Brittany.

"I don't have my glasses on. Some idiot put them over there where I can't reach. You'd think the hospital would hire people who could figure out that paralyzed people need things close." Mrs. Emerson spastically shoved at her overbed table as though she was trying to move it out of her way.

I reached over and found the glasses. "Hold on Mrs. Emerson, your glasses are filthy."

I took them into the bathroom and cleaned the lenses thoroughly. When I brought them back I handed them to Brittany and nodded for her to put them on Mrs. Emerson. Brittany placed them in Mrs. Emerson's shaking hands.

I whispered behind her head, "Help her get them on, Brittany."

Mrs. Emerson inspected us then spoke to Brittany. "You came in here yesterday afternoon didn't you."

Brittany nodded.

"Okay, you can stay. Hand me my watch."

"Brittany are you going to be okay now?"

"Yeah, I think so."

"I'll be back to check in on you. See you later Mrs. Emerson."

I knew Mrs. Emerson really needed to talk to someone, her anger clearly evident to my experienced ear. It was frustrating knowing that I would not have the time today and that Brittany, who was barely twenty years of age, would not have the insight to help her.

Rice was still waiting for me in the hallway. "We need to talk," she said. "Can we go sit somewhere privately?" She looked upset.

"Let's go back to the conference room."

When we were seated behind a closed door, Rice blurted out, "I don't want to be here. I don't like working with patients. I don't want to be a nurse. Do I have to stay?"

Normally I would have asked, "Are you sure?" Or perhaps convinced her to try it, just for today, but this was a sudden revelation only to her, not to Shelly or I. Rice appeared distraught.

"Let me go talk to the staff, Rice. I'll be back in a second."

I found Jackie who quickly assured me that they would reassume care for Rice's patient without hardship. I returned to Rice who at this point had begun to cry making visible lines in her blush. I pulled a tissue from my pocket.

"It's crinkled, but it's clean," I said, offering it to her.

"Thanks," she said, sniffling. She took a deep breath.

"You don't have to stay today, Rice. The staff will take care of your patient."

"I'm sorry to cause so much bother," she said between sobs.

"These things happen sometimes. It will work out." I put my arm around her shoulder and waited for her to speak.

"I've felt really strange these past few weeks, but I couldn't put my finger on it until this morning. I took one look at these patients and I felt nothing but disgust. I don't know how the nurses can do it."

"Nursing isn't for everyone Rice."

"But I really wanted to help people."

"There are other things besides nursing that you can do to help people."

"I feel so embarrassed."

"For what? Trying a career you thought you'd like? On the contrary, I have a lot of respect for you. What you did took guts. It's not easy to admit that you made a mistake."

"I think this is the hardest thing I've ever done in my life." She dabbed at her eyes again with the tissue. "So now what?"

"First you need to see the Director of the school and straighten out the paperwork. Then you need to go home and do some heavy duty thinking to figure out what it is you want to do next."

"I look at you. You are so lucky. You know what it is that you want. Everybody can see that you love what you do."

"But Rice, I'm not going to work here forever. I'm not sure what I'm going to do next." I said with a twinkle in my eye. "I don't know what I want to be when I grow up."

Rice's eyes had dried and she had even cracked a smile.

"You are going to be okay now Rice. I believe nursing is something you either love or hate. There's no middle ground. You don't need to make yourself miserable doing something you don't like. Life is hard enough without inducing misery!"

"I do feel as though a huge weight has been lifted off my shoulders," sighing deeply, "and yet I feel so guilty leaving my friends. We all worked so hard together. I feel like I'm letting them down."

"They'll understand. Trust me. There will be no hard feelings."

I heard the noisy rattling of the breakfast carts penetrating through the closed doors that made me check my watch.

"Rice, I've got to go check on everybody." I stood to leave.

"I'm sure you will find something that makes you happy. Make sure you stop back and let everybody know what you're up to. Good luck." I gave her a quick hug. Once I remembered that eight students were wandering about the floor unattended, I found it difficult to remain a focused supportive career counselor.

Loretta was the first to spot me as I emerged from the room.

"Karen, the breakfast tray just came and I'm in the middle of the bath. What should I do?" Her voice sounded distraught.

"Stop and think. What makes sense to you?"

"Would it be alright if I finished the bath first, then feed him?"

"Do you think that would be okay?"

"The food is in a warmer. It would probably wait. It would be easier for me to finish the bath first. I can make the bed later."

"Sounds like a good plan. Go with it."

Self-induced stress makes even the obvious difficult to see for some people on the first day.

Danielle had appeared on my left.

"My patient was lying in poop from his elbows to his toes. The aide helped me clean him up and change all the linen. Do you mind that she helped me?"

"Sounds like an appropriate use of resources."

"He's eating breakfast on his own, but the guy in the next bed needs help. Do you mind if I feed him?"

"That would be great. The staff will really appreciate it." I thought to myself, thank goodness I've got at least one strong student.

Amy moved into the spot vacated on my right.

"My patient is refusing a bath this morning. He says his wife will wash him when she comes in later this morning."

"Does he have his tray?"

"Yes."

"Did you help him set it up?"

"He didn't need help," Amy responded with confidence.

I knew the man had an IV in his hand, which would make opening the milk carton tricky.

"Come on," I said, "I haven't said hello to him yet."

I entered the room to find a man with greasy messy looking hair and several days of beard growth lying in a disheveled bed.

"Good morning, Mr. Smits, my name is Karen. I'm Amy's

instructor."

"Hello," he said. I watched as he struggled with the foil top on the juice cup.

"Boy the tops can be tricky sometimes, mind if I give you a hand?"

"Please do," he said. "This damn IV tubing makes it tough for me to maneuver."

"Would you like your toast buttered too?" I asked.

"If you don't mind."

I pulled the straw out of the wrapper and opened his napkin and put it on his chest. "It's tough to eat neatly lying in these beds, isn't it?"

"I always seem to dribble something down the front of me."

"Cream in your coffee?"

"Yes, please. I can never get those little buggers open."

"Mr. Smits, I understand that you prefer your wife to get you washed up."

"My wife comes in around 11 a.m. She helps if the nurses haven't gotten a chance to yet."

"Do you mind if Amy helps this morning?"

"No, not at all."

"Great then. We are all set. I'll check back with you guys later."

I winked at Amy as I left. "Don't forget the shave and shampoo," I whispered.

It is possible that Mr. Smits really had initially rejected Amy. It was also possible that as a novice, she had asked in a way that made Mr. Smits uncomfortable. But based on Shelly's earlier observations that she didn't trust Amy, I couldn't help but wonder what really had transpired. I made a note on my sheet, but for now extended her the benefit of the doubt.

Amy caught up with me halfway down the hall.

"I want you to know I really did ask him if I could help him with his tray and he refused."

"It happens sometimes Amy, especially if you are new."

Amy stood up straight, assuming an insulted pose. "I know how to set-up a patient's tray to eat. I worked as a nurse's aide once. He told me he could do it himself."

"Having an IV on a hand can make even the simplest chores

difficult. You have to try to anticipate the needs of your patients. I've noticed, especially with males, that asking for help is difficult. It threatens their ego. If you offer help for a specific task, in this case, opening a juice top, it is more likely to be accepted."

"You probably think I was trying to get out of his bath now too."

Interesting she should have asked that question in that manner. Perhaps out of guilt?

"Of course not," was my audible response. "It's fairly common for patients to refuse."

"But he didn't refuse you."

"It's all in how you ask. That's what I'm here for. Are you all set now?"

"Yes. I just wanted you to know I wasn't trying to get out of anything."

"Okay Amy."

She was slick. She knew just how to maneuver to recreate an incident to play to her favor. I could only hope that she would be a good nurse, because if she was a problem clinically, my documentation would have to be flawless to stick. I could tell by this first encounter that she was not one to accept correction or admit mistakes graciously.

I walked into Dale's room. Her patient looked very comfortable in a crisp linen bed. She was putting a ribbon in her patient's hair as I entered.

"Mrs. Goldman, you look lovely today."

"Dale is such a sweet girl," Mrs. Goldman responded. "She even did my nails," holding them out for me to see.

"We are going to walk next, right Mrs. Goldman?"

"If you say so sweetie," she responded, obviously enjoying the special attention.

Speaking to Dale I observed, "You look like you have everything in control here."

"It's easy to have only one. I have eight at work."

"Enjoy it."

"I would if I could get paid."

"Dream on," I said chuckling. "This is a hospital. Seriously though, do you need any help ambulating her?"

"The staff nurse said she was a one assist. She's so light I could carry her by myself if I needed to. I get three hundred pounders into a chair by myself at work."

"That's not a good idea for your back you know."

"I'm pretty strong," she said, displaying her bicep.

I decided that this was not a good time for a body mechanics lecture. After all, I was still trying to get Dale to relax around me.

"Normally, I like to be present when students get patients out of bed, but with all your experience, that seems unnecessary. Keep up the good work, Dale."

"Thanks," she said, looking surprised.

"You are lucky to have one of my best students today, Mrs. Goldman."

"I know," Mrs. Goldman said smugly.

As I left the room, I checked my list to see who I hadn't seen in awhile. I decided to check in on Russell. I peeked in Danielle's room as I passed. She was busy feeding an elderly gentleman, chatting away. We waved. The curtain was pulled around Russell's patient. A breakfast tray sat on the chair containing only a few crumbs of muffin. I checked under the curtain to see if it looked like Russell's shoes. It did. I knocked on the wall, simultaneously pretending to knock on the curtain.

"Russell?" I called.

"Nice trick," he said from behind the curtain. "I figured it was you."

"Is it safe for me to come in?"

"Yeah, Henry won't bite, will you?"

I came around the curtain. Russell was just preparing to begin his bath.

"Henry was an artillery man in WWII. He was just telling me about some pretty wild stuff," Russell explained.

"Hi, Mr. Talbot," I said, introducing myself.

"Call me Henry, please, or I will bite."

"Do you need me?" Russell asked.

"Nope. Just checking in. Did you find everything that you need?"

"Yup."

"Any questions?"

"Nope."

"Then carry on gentlemen," I saluted Mr. Talbot, then left

them alone to do their business.

Linda was across the hall. As I entered, she immediately got a relieved look on her face. "Can you help me with this lady? She needs to go to the bathroom, bad. I can't find a nurse and she's been calling for twenty minutes.

"Is she allowed to walk to the bathroom?"

"She said she was."

"Let me check the kardex first. What's her name?"

Linda looked at the name on the bed, "Little" she called.

I double checked the name on the chart outside the room and luckily found Mrs. Little's kardex on the cart where it was supposed to be. She was listed as bedside commode only. This meant she was allowed to use a portable seat with a built in potty right next to the bed. She had cancer that was spreading to her spine.

I grabbed a commode from the hallway and returned quickly, giving Linda instructions as we went. It turned out that Mrs. Little's strength faded quickly. She was barely able to support her own weight more than a few seconds.

"I'm glad I didn't walk her to the bathroom. She would never have made it," Linda remarked once in the hall.

"No kidding. That's why I never move a soul without checking first. How's Mrs. Pfizer?"

"I've got her washed up. I'm waiting for Dale to help me with the bed."

"Are you feeling more relaxed now?"

"Yeah," she responded enthusiastically. "This is fun! No offense, but clinical is a lot better than the labs."

"It's supposed to be."

Jackie put her head in. "Thanks for getting 19A on the commode. She's dead weight isn't she?" She didn't wait for a response. "I had to get 16B ready for Bone Marrow."

"Bone marrow? When are they doing that?"

"Dr. Fishbone just walked on the floor. He's great with students. I'm sure he wouldn't mind if they came in."

"How about the patient?"

"She probably won't mind, I'll go ask her."

Jackie briefly disappeared into the patient's room and reemerged holding up three fingers. "That's all that can fit in anyway. The room is tight."

"Linda, you are in the right place at the right time. You are about to see a bone marrow."

"Neat!" pausing a second, "What's a bone marrow?"

"Go find two more students that are available to go watch with you. I'll finish Mrs. Little and then meet you outside of 16B. In order to save time, I'll explain it when you are all together."

When I had Mrs. Little clean, comfortable and back on her chair, I hustled over to 16B. Danielle, Russell and Linda were waiting in the hallway.

"The doctor will be inserting a needle into bony tissue in order to obtain a sample of marrow. It is very interesting to watch, but keep in mind, it is a very scary and potentially painful procedure for the patient. When the blood is actually withdrawn from the marrow, some patients describe the pain as excruciating."

"Can't they anesthetize the area?" Linda asked.

"They use local anesthesia for the skin, and perhaps a sedative to help the patient relax, but there is no easy way to anesthetize the bone marrow."

"Why don't they use general anesthesia?" Russell asked.

"Too risky, plus there are a lot of side effects."

Jackie poked her head out, "He's starting."

"A couple of rules before you go in. One - Don't touch anything. Two - Don't back up without looking behind you. Three - In your excitement, don't forget that there is a patient under that sheet. Lastly - If you feel faint, leave the room promptly if there is time, or sit where you are if there isn't. Now skoot, you guys better get in there."

I headed back down the other wing, wondering what Loretta, Caitlin and Brittany were up to. I could see Brittany moving behind a closed curtain. I tiptoed in and saw her carefully forming a washcloth mitt and gently stroking Mrs. Emerson's leg in the proper direction. She did not see me. I left before she could. Students built confidence when they felt like they had done things on their own. As long as patient safety was maintained, I allowed them freedom to perform.

I could see Loretta at the foot of her patient's bed, folding a clean blanket gently over her feet. She was chatting politely with both her patient, a slender woman in her early 80's, and an early morning visitor. I poked my head casually around the half closed curtain and noticed that the left side rail was down and that the call bell was curled up on the wall, way beyond her patient's reach. I moved towards the side rail and pulled it up as I introduced myself to her patient.

"I've just had the most marvelous bath," the woman shared.

Loretta smiled, though obviously shaken from her instructor's discovery that she had broken a prime nursing commandment, thou shall never leave side rails down unattended.

"Are you a nurse too?" Mrs. Salem asked.

"Yes. I'm an RN."

"And you teach too?"

"Yes, sometimes I'm in a classroom and sometimes I'm here on the floors with you people."

"Isn't that marvelous," she said. "I always wanted to be a nurse. My mother wanted me to be a teacher."

"You were a teacher?"

"No, I dropped out of college and had 8 children, 17 grandchildren, and 3 great grandchildren," she said proudly.

"So you were a nurse and a teacher after all!"

"Don't you know it!" she replied.

Loretta had spotted the curled up call bell while I was chatting with her patient. I gave her a wink of approval as she fixed it. Suddenly, the woman began to cough uncontrollably. As I could hear the phlegm forming, I perfunctorily reached for the emesis basin and a wad of tissues while raising the head of the bed handing it to the patient, just in time. I recalled that she was here for an exacerbation of a lung disease commonly referred to as COPD. I checked her oxygen meter on the wall and readjusted it to the proper level, showing Loretta what I was doing as I worked. The episode lasted several minutes, during which Loretta seemed more stressed than the patient. When her respiratory pattern had returned to normal, the woman patted Loretta's hand.

"It looks worse than it really is, sweetheart."

I pulled my stethoscope from around my neck. "Mind if I listen?"

"Be my guest dear. Everyone else does. They tell me I'm

interesting. Beats me, I'd rather listen to the Grand Ole Opry."

I checked her lungs. "Your heart's got a great country beat. Ever consider having this recorded?"

Mrs. Salem, proud of her special heart, invited several other students who had entered the room to listen as I explained the various sounds they were hearing. Back in the hall I asked Amy what she needed.

"Nothing, I'm all finished. Is there anything else you want me to do?"

"Boy you are quick. Before you do that, let's go see Mr. Smits again."

"His wife is there now."

"So, let's go visit Mr. and Mrs. Smits then."

Amy shrugged her shoulders and sighed. She followed me begrudgingly. From the doorway, I could see Mrs. Smits straightening out Mr. Smits toiletries to put them away.

"I left them out so he could reach them easily," Amy said quickly.

"Did you forget to shave Mr. Smits?" I asked. The fuzzy face was obvious even from a distance.

"His wife came in just as I was about to or I would have done it. I thought I was supposed to give them privacy. I can ask him," she said in a tone of mock respect, "if that's what you think I should do."

"Amy, the clinical assignment this morning was to give AM hygiene. That includes a shave for male patient who cannot do so without assistance. Apparently no one has done it for days. So what do you think you should do today? It's only 1O a.m. We have another hour before we leave."

Instead of answering me, Amy turned and headed towards her patient. I left her to find her own way. Clearly, Amy would not be calling me her favorite instructor this semester. When patient care is questionably given, I am no student's friend. On the way back down the hall, I passed Rita, the hospital's Patient Representative. We stopped and chatted amicably for a few moments.

"What brings you here today, Rita?"

"Do you know anything about Mr. Peters?"

"My student has him. I know his history."

"I need to try and talk to him. Apparently the family has some concerns about his progress."

"I'll go with you. I was on my way in there anyway to check on my student."

Fortunately, I was several steps ahead of Rita. I entered the room, took one look, then did an abrupt about face, stopping Rita in her tracks.

"Give us a minute if you don't mind Rita," I stammered. "Uhh, he's not in a position to chat."

"Sure," she said in an unsuspecting voice. "I have two others on this floor to see anyway."

I shut the door behind her, just in case. Mr. Peters was lying stark naked on the bare mattress. I grabbed the nearest sheet and covered the poor man. Despite my shock and horror, I somehow managed to keep my voice slow and quiet.

"What in the blazes is going on here?"

Caitlin looked like a deer caught in headlights. If I had said what I was really thinking, she was sure to start crying.

"Let's get some sheets under him quickly. You can explain later."

With me leading the way, we were able to return Mr. Peters bed to a normal state in record time. I was just tucking in the final corner when Rita entered.

"Everything okay in here?" Rita looked over at Caitlin, who was still ashen.

"We are all set now," I answered, slightly short of breath. "I thought you had two other patients to see."

"They were both off the floor for tests. Is Mr. Peters up for talking?"

"He'll nod yes and no. The staff said he has been kind of out of it since he came in." I loaded my arms with the soiled linens and signaled to Caitlin to follow me out of the room. "All yours Rita," I said non chalantly. "By the way, his hearing is better on the left."

I took Caitlin to the conference room, reminding myself to count to ten before speaking.

"You're really upset with me aren't you?" she asked when I reached about seven.

"I just don't understand what I saw. Do you have any idea

who that lady was?"

"No."

"She is the hospital's patient representative. She came to talk with Mr. Peters because his family is concerned about the care he's getting. If I hadn't stopped her, we would be in hot water right now."

So much for counting to ten.

"I'm not really sure why what I did wrong, though from your response I could tell it was bad."

"What possessed you to take all the linens off the bed?"

"He was incontinent of stool and I couldn't figure out how to put the clean sheets on without messing them up. So I figured I would take off the dirty ones first, wash him, then put the clean ones back on."

"Why was he naked?"

"He soiled his gown. I was just getting ready to put a new one on when you walked in."

I was speechless.

"The mannequins in the lab never soiled a bed," she said in her defense.

"True," I said beginning to soften. I knew I would find this funny someday.

"He was only like that for less than a minute," she added.

"How about if I show you the preferred method to change dirty linen?"

"I think you'd better."

Caitlin and I were in the linen room discussing soiled beds when Linda interrupted us.

"Karen, you better come quickly. Russell just passed out."

"Oh no," already running down the hall. "Did he hit anything?"

"No," called Linda, lagging behind.

Russell was on the floor, leaning against the wall outside of the curtained area. Danielle was at his side. Russell was pale and obviously embarrassed.

"Are you okay?"

"I tried to make it to the hall," he sighed. "Sorry."

"It happens."

Behind the curtain in 16B, I could hear screams of agony.

Danielle went back to the patient and reassumed holding her hand as I helped Russell out of the room to a chair in the hallway.

"I can't believe I did this."

"Did you eat breakfast this morning?"

"Yeah. It was just really hot in there. When she started screaming I started to lose it. I'm going to make a lousy nurse if I can't handle stuff like that."

"Actually, I'm glad to find out that you are human. There were rumors, you know."

"You shouldn't believe what you hear."

"Seriously though, that's what happens when you have a heart. If nothing ever bothered you, you wouldn't be very empathetic toward the patients. Besides, it can happen to the best of us."

"Right," he said unbelieving.

"At least I made it to the hallway before I passed out when I saw my first bone marrow aspiration."

"Really?"

"Believe me, it gets easier, but some things still are tough to watch. The more painful for the patient, the harder it is for me to watch. The smell of burning flesh from the electro-cautery in the operating room made me pass out when I was a student."

"What did you do?"

"Became a medical-surgical floor nurse instead!"

Linda and Danielle joined us in the hallway.

"Russell don't feel bad," Linda told him. "I almost went down right before you did when the needle started grinding into the bone. Remember when I left saying I needed to get a kleenex?"

Danielle joined in, "That was like ancient evil torture. Boy I really felt for that lady."

I checked my watch again. It was 1O:4O already. Clinical was scheduled to end at 11:00. I had eight charts to review and one more set of rounds to make.

"Are you guys done with everything?" I asked everyone as Dale joined our group. "You need to check side-rails, call bells, get your patients turned and then let me check your charting."

Linda looked at her watch. "Oh no, I still have to make my bed."

Danielle and Dale offered Linda assistance and headed off, agreeing to help turn each others' patients once Linda's was finished.

Russell assured me that he was fine and that he just need to finish charting on Harry.

During my final rounds, I complimented Amy on Mr. Smits clean shaven face and tidy room. My review of her charting revealed that she had forgotten to record the amount of liquids Mr. Smits had consumed at breakfast. Other sections on the chart had been left totally blank.

"I told the nurse and she said she would write it on the sheet," Amy countered.

"We are expected to do this," as I dragged Amy back to the chart board to complete the days tasks. "Let me show you so you'll know for next week."

As I played a losing game of beat the clock, the students began to gather around me like bees returning to the nest.

"If you all bring me your charts, I'll be able to check them quicker."

Danielle, Russell and Dale had completed their charts accurately. Caitlin had charted the breakfast intake for 9 p.m. instead of a.m. When I pointed it out, she scribbled out the error before I could stop her.

"This is a legal document Caitlin. In class you were taught how to correct errors using one line to cross it out."

"Oh, I forgot. Do I need a new one?"

"The staff has already charted on this. I'll fix it, you watch."

After correcting Caitlin's errors and teaching her how to properly document the information, it was now 11:26.

"Are we having post-conference today?" Russell asked.

"There is no time. You all need to be in class by 12:00. Once I've checked your chart, get going or you'll miss lunch."

Loretta had several questions, some of which I deferred for the time being, suggesting instead that she join me on the walk back to the school building. Linda had left several areas on her charts blank waiting for me to confirm that she was doing it right. After she was set, I went quickly from room to room, stopping to gather my post-it "Freshman Student" notes and stuff them into my pockets. I peeked in each of our rooms to check to see if we had left the patients safe and comfortable in their beds, with the rooms in proper order. I was pleased to see that even Caitlin's room was acceptable and that her patient was positioned comfortably on his side. He looked a lot better with clothes on.

I retrieved my coat from the staff locker room and as I tossed it over my arm, a whiff of smoke filled my nose, evidence that not all staff adhered to the non-smoking policy.

"Lucky you, going home already," an aide said.

"I wish I were. I have to teach class now."

"Oh. Are you guys here tomorrow?"

"No. The students have lab all day tomorrow. We will see you next week."

"Oh."

The tone of her response revealed that she didn't have a clue as to what the nursing faculty did all week. From her vantage point, it appeared non-taxing. I caught Jackie in the station as I walked past.

"Call me if we missed anything."

"Thanks for all your help. Your students were great. They're always a big help."

"They didn't bug you too much?"

"No, not at all. Hardly knew they were here. See you next week!"

When I reached the elevators, Loretta was waiting for me. She asked a zillion questions while we walked back to my office. Upon arrival, I checked my watch. I had two minutes to eat lunch and get to class. I grabbed my sandwich and began to chew it while I gathered my lecture notes and handouts. I checked the mirror as I passed. My hair was messy and barely any make-up remained from the 5:3O a.m. application. No time to correct it, I headed out the door passing Shelly as I rounded the bend.

"How did it go today?" I asked turning and walking backwards down the narrow hallway.

"Did three shampoos this morning," she reported, "how about you?"

"Had enough trouble just getting them dressed. Catch you after class," I called as I approached the stairwell to descend to the basement level classrooms.

As I shoved the last, rather large bite of sandwich into my

mouth I entered a gauntlet of students lining the hallways in mixed attire.

"You're late," one dared to say.

I choked down my final bite then countered with, "It's Loretta's fault."

"I'm here, you can't blame me!" Loretta piped up.

"How long do we have to wait for an instructor here?" another voice asked.

"Well, I was an Associate Professor in my last job, so I guess you'll have to give me thirty minutes."

I struggled to find the correct key on my janitorial looking ring. As the old door opened, we were met with a blast of heat, courtesy of an old building remiss of temperature controls.

"This is going to be fun today," I said sarcastically as I entered the steamy room, opened a window and turned on the air conditioner to duke it out with the relentless radiator.

Fortunately the two hour lecture was on a topic that lended itself to anecdotal stories that kept the students alert despite the warm room and inadequate sleep. By 1:58, students began to gather their belongings while I spoke, indicating that a late dismissal today would not be tolerated. I finished the content quickly for my benefit, well aware that at this point it was falling on deaf, exhausted ears. The closing of my notebook was a signal that required no explanation.

A few students left quickly, headed for their full or part time evening jobs, a self inflicted tortuous schedule. Several students remained after class, some wanted to share their morning experiences, some wanted assistance with clinical paperwork, and the remainder just wanted to not miss anything that I might say. Being surrounded by nursing students thirsty for knowledge simultaneously invigorated and exhausted me mentally.

By 2:3O I had had it.

"It's been a long day for all of us. What do you say we head home?"

One student looked at her watch, grabbed her books and started for the door. "I've got to catch a school bus, see ya!"

We all gathered our gear and with loaded arms, headed upstairs to leave. I had finally shaken loose from all the students by the time I reached the solitude of my office. I opened the door and collapsed on my desk chair, then threw my throbbing feet up on the desk.

"Ahhh," said it all.

I pulled out a pad to finish my notes on the students' clinical performance from the morning. I had written one name when six students entered my office.

"No rest for the weary?" I pleaded.

"We heard Rice left. Is there anything we could do to help her stay?"

"That's a very nice gesture, but it's not fair for me to discuss it with you."

"We understand."

"Is she okay?" one gal asked, not to be put off so easily.

"She's fine, really. She'll probably call you when she's ready to talk about it."

"I hope it wasn't anything we said or did," said another.

"I wouldn't worry about that. I'd worry about next week's assessment validation," attempting to change the subject.

The students took the hint and after asking a multitude of questions about the next validation, they finally left. By the time I finished writing notes from the morning clinical, prepared a mountain of materials for the next morning's 7:30 a.m. lab, and checked my E-mail, it was pushing 4:30.

I pulled the eight clinical care plan folders the students had turned in from my tote bag and stacked them on my desk. Review of these, if done properly, represented hours of work. Yet, the more corrections and comments I made, the faster the students got the hang of them, making them easier and quicker to review. I half-peeked at Danielle's, hoping that maybe I'd get at least one good one the first clinical week. It looked okay. I didn't dare look at some of the others. It would be too depressing after a long day.

I looked around at the stacks of papers scattered across the desk. I had an endless array of "to do" projects awaiting my attention. There were all kinds of things that would make a lecture more interesting or demonstration more effective.

Eventually, I would get to each stack, between exams or while Shelly taught, or when I wasn't inundated with students or reviewing care plans. Maybe tomorrow, maybe at the end of the semester, maybe some weekend or evening at home if I was in the mood. Since all of these projects were my ideas anyway, no one really cared when or if I actually did them. But I would be haunted by a nagging sense of incompleteness 24 hours a day until I did. My own insatiable desire to constantly improve was the driving force against which my sensibilities were powerless.

I began to shuffle through one pile when the phone rang, breaking through the serenity of the empty office and halls. My latch key kids were fighting and wanted to know when I'd be home. My concentration shattered, I decided to call it a day.

"I'm on my way now guys," I told the kids, "I'm putting my coat on as we speak."

I stood up and hung up the phone. I stared at the desk blankly for a minute then grabbed a few care plans and shoved them in my bag, just in case I had free time at home that evening. Between the kids, house chores, and husband, that was highly unlikely, but taking stuff home with me was a hard habit to break. Still standing by my desk, I caught a glimpse of a new handout in progress. I added a few words to it, then tossed the paper in my bag to go home with the others.

"Enough!" I said to myself. "It will still be here tomorrow."

Leaving the messy desk intact, I turned out my office light and slowly began to close the door. I paused at midpoint and leaned against the door jam. I looked around the tiny room.. at the samples of new equipment being introduced on the clinical units that was collecting in corners around the room.. at the countless textbooks and reference books that overflowed from the shelves, some worn edged favorites and others still pristine, calling out to be read... and at the nursing mementos, gifts from appreciative past students whose lives I had touched. This room overflowed with vital pieces of my identity as a nurse, the career I had grown to love.

Driving home, I reflected that it was a good day by instructor standards. No one died, no one killed anyone, no one dropped anyone, no one made any life threatening mistakes and we didn't forget to do anything really major. I chastised myself for not checking to see if Linda really bathed her patient and couldn't quite recall seeing if Russell had remembered to turn his patient today, but there are just so many places you can be at one time.

At a stop light, I wrote a note to myself to check Linda and Russell next week and shoved it into my notebook. I decided to keep the pen close in case I thought of something else before the light changed. I usually did.

In a few moments, the peace and quiet would slowly dissipate and like a chameleon, I would assume my other roles as wife and mother. I measured contentment with my job by comparing it to a three mile run. Often, runs start out with a feeling like you get the chance to "run away" from everything that is stressing you. At some point in the run, the stress is relieved and you begin running back. The sooner you want to start running back, the more contentment you have.

"Yes, tomorrow," I thought, smiling. "I'll be back."

"When God gives any man wealth and possessions, and enables him to enjoy them, to accept his lot and be happy in his work this is a gift of God. He seldom reflects on the days of his life, because God keeps him occupied with gladness of heart."

Ecclesiastes 5: 19-20

18

Teaching with Passion

I was often asked during my seventeen years of teaching if I missed nursing. I definitely didn't miss working the odd shifts or holidays away from home, but I can't say that I ever got a chance to miss nursing. I did some of my best nursing from the sidelines.

As an instructor, I had the freedom to choose whatever level of involvement with the staff and patients I desired. While many of my colleagues elected a strictly supervisory role, I preferred jumping into the trenches with my students. I spent a lot of time in the patient's rooms assisting or observing my students. As a result, I got very involved with the patients that we took care of week after week. There was always something we would think of to improve the patient's care. Patient advocacy became my favorite pastime on the units.

Over the course of each semester, the students would gradually improve and become more self-directed. I found that I had pockets of time to spare. Although hanging out in the conference room grading papers was one option, that wasn't my style. So here I was, a master's prepared Medical-Surgical Clinical Specialist wandering "free lance" on a floor filled with needy patients, eager as a racehorse at the gate. It never took long to find a place where I was needed. I'm not talking beds or baths either. Hospital administration generally provided adequate staff for these measurable services. I'm talking about the non-billable fluff that makes the difference in people's lives.

There were patient teaching opportunities everywhere. People who didn't understand their disease. Pre-ops who didn't understand what was going to happen. Post-ops who didn't understand what had been done. Diabetics who needed help with insulin shots. Patients headed home for discharge not knowing what caused their illness. The physicians were required by law to explain things to patients as part of obtaining the consent.

Unfortunately, patients commonly misunderstood the doctor's explanation. Sometimes it was due to just one confusing word or the lack of a visual image to make it clear.

* * *

"Karen, my man in 11-A is going home this morning," Russell began.

"11-A...Remind me. What's his diagnosis?" I had fourteen patients to keep track of that day.

"Prostate surgery. He had a TURP (essentially a roto-rooter of the prostate done via the urethra of penis)."

"He's going home already?" Insurance companies had trimmed the previous standard five to six day stays to three days, but the man in 11-A was post-op from yesterday.

"They are sending him home with the catheter in."

I rolled my eyes as I reviewed all the possible complications that could occur at home. Not all the changes in medicine these days were in the patient's best interest.

"He's going to need some teaching before he goes."

Russell stood tall and proud and grinned from ear to ear. The student knew he'd earn brownie points knowing how much I valued patient education and independent thinking.

"I taught him about his catheter, how to use the leg bag and switch to the night bag. I got him all the supplies he will need."

"Kegel's?" I asked, referring to the perineal exercises that would help him regain continence.

"Done already," he said, beaming.

"Good for you! What do you need me for?"

"He was asking me questions I couldn't answer. I told him that my instructor could help. He's waiting for you."

The man in 11-A was lying in bed fully dressed with his suitcase opened on the chair. I introduced myself. He went to sit up, but hesitated at the halfway point.

"I'm more tired than I thought. Just getting dressed wiped me out," he looked me over and smiled. "Your student told me that you knew everything about my surgery."

"Thanks for putting the pressure on me Russell," I said to my student.

After a few questions, I realized that this 65 year old man in 11-A didn't understand the basic anatomical location of his prostate. He had been too embarrassed to tell his surgeon.

"After all," he said, "a guy should know where his guy stuff is, right?"

I grabbed a brown paper towel from the bathroom to draw on and commenced class. As usual, two other students joined midway through my pocket paper lecture. It took less than five minutes to turn a confused intelligent man into an active knowledgeable participant in his own care.

Later while I was in the med room watching another student, I saw the man in 11-A walking up the hall to go home, accompanied by a friend carrying his suitcase. He stopped, pulled a folded brown paper towel out of his pocket and waved it at me mouthing the word "thanks".

In my mind I thought, "No charge!" Once again, it was the intangible, non-reimbursable needs of the patient that were most imperative.

* * *

The first time I saw her, she was in the hall crying. The woman was in her forties, slender, nice looking with conservative dress. Her husband was being attended to by a multitude of nurses. From my post in the hall near the cart where Linda and Caitlin were preparing medications for my approval, I could see a man sitting up in bed with a tube protruding from his nose, holding an emesis basin, retching. The nurse attending him quickly drew the curtain, blocking my view.

Perhaps because they were a younger couple, or maybe because his wife was so involved with his care, I was told not to take him as a patient by the staff. I really didn't know what was wrong with him. I assumed cancer since it was an oncology floor.

When the wife had gathered herself and looked up, our eyes met. I smiled at her in a way that simultaneously expressed concern. She smiled back, accepting the unspoken support. That was the extent of our relationship. The students and I had no responsibility towards him. And yet, week after week, his wife and I shared the hallway.

"How's he doing today?" I began to ask, still clueless as to his problems.

She'd stop and chat with me, seemingly eager to share her pain with someone, anyone. My face had become as familiar to her as the other fixtures on the wall in the hall. She wanted her husband home for the holidays and was hoping that we would get him well enough to be able to handle it. It was early November.

She watched me field a myriad of questions from students and staff and began to use me in the same way. I taught her about the IV equipment as she prepared to take him home. I defined terms, explained procedures, or addressed whatever her needs were that day. Still, in respect of patient privacy laws, I had not read his chart.

At this point, I wasn't sure why the staff still didn't want students to take care of him. Since students had only one or two patients, they had time to provide extra comforts and attention and were always well prepared. As students, they were double-checked on all their medications and as a result we often discovered things that should be corrected, like unsafe medication combinations or medication orders that had expired.

The man was transferred to a hospital in Boston with high hopes for treatment, but returned, discouraged and as sick as ever. A week later, he was made a Hospice patient. One day, I asked the wife if she would mind having a student.

"I think that would be nice," she replied.

Reading the chart nearly brought me to tears. He had been not feeling right for about a year. He had sought medical attention promptly, but all the early exams were read as negative. Nine months after the initial tests, he was diagnosed with intestinal cancer that had spread widely via the mesentery, the blood network that supplies all the intestines. It was inoperable and the cancer was not responding to any of the chemo regimes. A review of the earlier tests revealed a shadow on the intestine where it initially started. Human eyes had missed it because it was not easy to see... then.

My careful review of the chart revealed that the man had not been receiving adequate nutrition. His plain IV bags brought him fluid and about 500 calories a day, with no vitamins, minerals or protein. He had not eaten any food in weeks that had stayed down.

I assigned Linda to take care of him. During pre-conference, we decided to make "improved nutrition" the goal for the day.

Linda was prepared to discuss it with the physician. I spoke to the wife, asking her what they had discussed concerning her husband's nutritional needs.

"Nothing. I asked them if he needed something more for energy, but they said that's why they kept him on IVs."

"Did you know that he's only getting about 500 calories a day?"

"No, really? That explains it. I've been wondering why he's lost so much weight. He can barely stand he's so weak. He vomits everything he tries to eat. What more could they do?"

I told her about hyper-alimentation, a high power IV solution that was a complete diet. "That might give him some strength back. The cancer cells are much better competitors when nutrition stores are meager. He needs enough to give the normal cells a chance."

"I know it can't save him. Nothing can," she went on quietly, "you know the chemo didn't work."

I nodded.

"If he could only have his strength back enough to get home for Christmas."

I suggested she speak with her doctor and the hospice nurse. Hospice patients were often withdrawn from life prolonging treatments unless they were being used for the purpose of providing comfort. It was uncomfortable for this man to be so weak, a valid argument. My student was poised and ready to approach the doctors, but unfortunately, they didn't come on our shift.

The next day, I found the wife early in our shift.

"The doctor wouldn't go for it," she told me looking discouraged. "I had a really long talk with him and really tried to change his mind about it, but he was vehemently opposed to it."

"Why?" I asked, incredulous.

"He said it won't make a difference at this point," sighing. "He said he would increase his potassium in the IV."

"That will help, but that's not nutrition."

"He must have thought I was stupid. I know we need more calories. I really wish we had done something sooner. The hospice nurse thought the hyper-alimentation was a good idea too, but wouldn't disagree with the physician."

Later that day, I helped the man from the commode back to bed. He was skin and bones. He couldn't get his pants up alone because he was feeling weak and dizzy. A proud man, he was humiliated to have to be helped. The picture of a robust looking couple taken on a hike from last year's vacation sitting on the bedstand behind him was haunting. Vomiting daily for six weeks without adequate nutrition took its toll long before the cancer would have. When the man could no longer walk to the bathroom on his own accord, he lost his will to live. We had been too late and not nearly nosey enough to help. Who knows? Maybe he could have made home for one last Christmas.

* * *

"Now that's my idea of a perfect patient! Sterile dressings on both feet and hips, an infected chest wound, plus a triple lumen (IV that went into her chest) that will need to be flushed on our time and IV antibiotics."

"Don't forget that Dorrie's also on isolation," the staff nurse added.

"Icing on the cake!"

I was always on the lookout for complicated patient situations that would allow me to offer the students a multitude of experiences. I peeked in to catch a glimpse of Dorrie as the nurse, wearing a mask and gown, entered for her morning care. I couldn't see much. Dorrie was curled up like a huge turtle on the bottom half of the bed.

"Can you give me a boost?" the nurse called, seeing me stand idle.

I looked down at my outfit, a dressy print skirt and long sleeved white taffeta blouse, appropriate for the afternoon lecture, but not patient care.

"Hang on," I replied. I found another isolation gown and mask stored in the cabinet outside the door and quickly covered up my good clothes. I entered the room, barely large enough for her bed, grabbed some gloves and took the side closest to the door.

"Dorrie, we're going to pull you up in bed," the nurse explained.

Dorrie grunted a reply. The nurse looked at me.

"On three."

The large turtle weighed a ton. No sooner did we pull her up in bed, she curled herself back into a ball, basically returning herself to the position she started in.

"Oh well. Want to try again?" I asked the nurse.

"I don't know. Let me check her oxygen level first."

She slipped the oximeter on Dorrie's finger to take a reading.

"Oxygen level is fine. Leave her. I'll get her up later. Thanks anyway."

I went back to making out my clinical assignment for the next day. Dorrie did not seem like a very communicative patient, so I assigned her to Amy since she was a less dynamic student in need of dressings and IV experience. I generally saved my better communicators or all round stars for the patient's who were in need of more emotional support, like the young mother just diagnosed with terminal cancer across the hall.

Reviewing Dorrie's chart, I discovered that she was a long-term diabetic, which explained her leg ulcers. She had chronic lung disease, secondary to a long history of smoking, which she gave up several years prior. Her lung disease was being controlled by steroids, which explained the large moon face I had seen, albeit briefly, the hump on her back and the truncal obesity that created the turtle-like appearance. She had undergone open heart surgery about six weeks ago in another hospital, which explained how she got the chest wound.

She was in our hospital because when she came for a doctor's appointment, she had a respiratory arrest in her car in the parking lot. Someone spotted her slumped over and she was resuscitated. The chest wound developed a serious bacterial infection while recovering in ICU. She was eventually transferred to our medical ward for long term IV antibiotics.

According to the social history, Dorrie had no children and lived alone in an apartment. She didn't look very independent now.

The first week of clinical, I barely saw Dorrie. I came only in time to intercept horrendous sterile dressing technique being used by my borderline student, Amy. Throughout the procedure, Dorrie was quiet, patient, and somewhat complacent. Dorrie's sheets were messy and hair unkempt, both common telltale signs that the morning care was not done.

When questioned, the student said, "I did as much as she would let me. She slept through the whole bath and refused to let me comb her hair. The nurse said to change the sheets once she was in the chair."

I couldn't imagine what a chore getting this patient up would be like. The dressings took an hour to finish. I realized from the line of students outside the door that our morning session was nearing closure. Upon leaving, I apologized to the staff nurse that we didn't have time to get Dorrie out of bed.

"No problem. You got all the dressings done. Getting her up is the easy part."

"Sure," I thought.

The next week, Dorrie's physician notes revealed a definitive diagnosis of osteomyelitis of the ribs next to her chest wound. Osteomyelitis is a severe bone infection that can result in destruction of the bone unless prolonged antibiotic therapy is able to control it. Dorrie was infected with a particularly virulent and persistent organism, complicated further by her decreased natural resistance thanks to the diabetes. The consulting physician felt her only chance of healing was to surgically remove the infected bone. The surgery would need to be done at another hospital. According to the note, Dorrie was apparently undecided as to what to do.

Bill, her nurse for the day, managed to have her less disheveled looking when I arrived to watch the dressings. He skillfully changed the dressings over the deep leg wounds with the same degree of sensitivity exhibited towards the mannequins used in the practice lab.

"Miss Holmes, are you comfortable?" As a sign of respect, I preferred calling patients older than myself by their proper names unless they requested otherwise. She was lying on her side, head scrunched up near the side rails.

"I'm okay," she said in a quiet little voice.

"Does your leg hurt at all?"

"I don't feel a thing. I guess that is why I've got the problem to begin with."

"Gently now," I said to the student. I moved up towards the head of the bed so I could see Dorrie's face and for the first time, saw her as a person, not a collection of nursing skills handy for practice.

"How long has your leg been like this?"

She looked down at her ankle.

"Oh, about a year. The one on my hip is new. Got that while I was laid up for the heart surgery last month. This one on my chest scares me."

"From what I read on your chart, I understand you might need surgery."

"Some doctors came in and told me I needed surgery. One talked so fast, I couldn't understand half of what he said. Another one was there too, but she didn't speak English too well. They asked me if I had any questions then left before I could think of them."

"That's frustrating isn't it," amazed at how aware and communicative this lady really was.

"It's not like I can get up and run after them."

My student interrupted with a question about technique. I answered it then went back to Dorrie and kneeled down where her head was still pressed to the bars.

"Are you sure you're comfortable?" I asked again.

"I'm really fine," she said looking inquisitively at me. "You say you read my chart?"

"Yes. What can I help you with?"

Dorrie proceeded with an entourage of questions about her illness and the impending surgery.

"Do you think I should have the surgery?"

"I think you need to talk with the surgeons and explore all your options. Talking with them is not a commitment. Decide after you have all the facts."

My busy week flew by. I'm sure to Dorrie, lying in that bed, it dragged endlessly.

When "today's" student, Dale, began the arduous chore of changing Dorrie's dressing, I assumed my post near Dorrie's head to keep her company and distracted.

"How are you doing, Mrs. Holmes?" I asked once in position. This social greeting, seldom answered in passing took on new meaning when used at the bedside with full eye contact.

"They can't operate. My heart won't make it."

"I saw that in your chart. That must have been tough to hear."

"I had really wrestled with the idea of the surgery to begin with. But once I realized that taking the infected bone out was my only chance to cure this, I was ready. Now..."she stared off into space as several minutes went by.

"I see you made yourself a no-code," I said breaking the silence. "That was a pretty brave thing to do."

Dale looked at me, shocked that I would raise such a sensitive topic.

"I've been ill like this for over a year." She looked around at her tiny room, the narrow window that offered a view of the hospital delivery dock, and the closed door that protected other patients from her infection but sealed her fate of solitary confinement. "This is not living. This is some kind of hellish torture. If I die, I don't need them bringing me back for more of this. I don't know why I didn't just die already."

The words Dorrie spoke struck a chord deep in my soul. This turtle woman had no purpose for living. Her quiet acceptance of the pain, discomfort and solitary confinement had made her easy for us nurses to ignore. We had written her off as a non-entity, as though she was a non-responsive patient with only basic physical needs. That would soon change. After all, I had eight students hanging around who were required to do whatever I told them.

We adopted Dorrie as our project. For the next couple of weeks she got my best students. We washed her hair, primped her and lavished her with our attention. When we figured out that she liked to sleep in until 9:30 or 10:00, generally unthinkable in a hospital, we left her undisturbed and then reheated her breakfast when she woke up. When she was taken off of the strict isolation precautions, I would use her room as my final post for the day, which assured her visits from all the students. As the weeks passed, Dorrie flourished, regained strength and even began ambulating in the hallway.

She hung up the phone as I entered.

"I'm sorry Miss Holmes. I didn't mean to intrude."

"You're not. Come in," she beckoned with her hand. "I'm not getting anywhere anyway." Her eyes filled with tears.

I went over, sat down next to her and put my gloveless hand on her shoulder. I didn't have to ask what was wrong.

"They've told me I can't go home again. I live on the third

floor of an apartment. There is no elevator."

I sat quietly while she sobbed a few moments then blew her nose.

"It so difficult to try and close out an apartment from this bed. My furniture... my pictures... my papers. There are so many things that I'll never see again." She paused again to blow her nose. "I've been trying to tell my cousin what to do with everything. I hate to be a burden to her. I've been on the phone all morning making arrangements to empty out the apartment so she doesn't have to do it all." She reached for another tissue. "No one should have to go through this."

Dorrie's suffering was palpable. As she laid there, with sores on her legs, wound on her chest, weakened lungs, and now stripped of all her personal treasures, all I could think of was Job. This helpless woman, riddled with incapacitating diseases that had spared her mind, experienced the full throws of the final insult of degradation that comes with the loss of independence.

Her grief was intense and needed an outlet. She repeated her story over and over to anyone who would listen as though by doing so this involuntary lifestyle change might make some sense to her. Eventually we talked about nursing homes, the myths that formed the basis for some of her fears and the realities from my own experiences. Given her situation, a nursing home actually offered an opportunity for the social interactions that hospitalization could not provide. Over the years, this conversation had become familiar to me, although the faces were all different. I might ease a mind or allay some fears, but I could never remove the emotional pain of the stark reality of a body that has timed out. Intuitively, we all know that "someday" it will be our time. For Dorrie, "someday" had come and it was not easy.

The following week, Dale pulled me away from a crowd of students.

"Karen, come quick! It's Dorrie."

I bolted down the hall expecting the worst. Of all days, this was the first week we hadn't taken Dorrie for a patient since everyone had taken her once already. Dorrie was lying flat on her back. Danielle was holding her eyelids open while Jackie, the staff nurse, was showering them with saline from a syringe. Dorrie's eyes were reddened beyond bloodshot.

"What happened?"

Danielle explained, "She accidentally put room deodorizer drops in her eyes instead of artificial tears."

The how and why would be sorted out later.

"Ohhh this hurts," Dorrie moaned loudly.

"We need a better way to do this," Jackie said, looking to me for suggestions.

"I'll be right back," as I hurried to the supply room, Dale in tow. "Go see what she can have for pain."

I grabbed an IV bag of Normal Saline and tubing from the supply cart. I assembled the IV as I hurriedly walked back to the room and gave it to Jackie to use as a gentler flush.

Linda and Caitlin were holding Dorrie's hand and keeping her distracted from her pain.

Dale had returned with the medication sheets. I was proud of my students performing as a team for the first time.

A physician who was making rounds on the floor, entered and took control. He was a neurologist, not an opthamologist, so proceeded carefully outside of his element.

"Keep flushing," he said as he looked at her eyes from the end of the bed. "What did she put in her eyes?"

Danielle handed him the bottle. "I just stopped by to say hello and noticed her eyes were bright red. I called in the nurse as soon as I realized what happened. The real eye drops were in her drawer."

"How about some pain medication, doctor?" I asked.

"She has an order for Demerol prn," Dale read. "She sure looks like she could use some."

But the "doctor" preferred to wait on pain medication until he checked out the suggested treatment for the deodorizer. It took over twenty minutes, three gentle reminders and one plea for the humanity of the situation before the "doctor" finally relinquished with a "oh go ahead and give her something." This was yet another potent reminder of a "nurses" place in the hierarchy of medicine and the consequence of my decision twenty years earlier.

When we checked on Dorrie before we left for the day, she was sound asleep, back in turtle position.

We were not scheduled to be on the unit the next day, but I

couldn't get Dorrie out of my mind. I kept visualizing her moaning, eyes spread open while bag after bag of fluid was flushed across the irritated surface of her eyes. I wanted to bring her something. A survival reward.

I was drawn to a stash of brand new unused teddy bears I had in my closet. Each teddy bear was about 15 inches tall, blonde, and had a medal around its neck. I chastised myself for thinking this an acceptable gift for a grown woman in her seventies. I put it back twice as I debated its appropriateness. I was too tired to go to the store, so I eventually stuffed one in a gift bag, covered it with tissue, and brought it anyway, figuring I didn't have to bring it to her if I changed my mind.

I waited until lunchtime to go up to the floor. Several of the nursing staff spotted me.

"Karen, what are you doing up here today?"

"Can't get enough of you!" I replied. "How's Dorrie?"

"Her eyes are really red, but she can see. Thanks to your quick thinking student."

Dorrie was sitting in a chair and smiled when she saw me walk in. I pouted my lower lip out.

"Mrs. Holmes, I felt so bad for you yesterday. How are you doing?"

"That was the most horrible experience of my life. I thought I had seen it all. That was so painful. When they were putting the water in my eyes it felt as though they were rubbing sand against them. It was awful."

Oh what the heck, I thought, pulling the gift from behind my back. "I brought you a little something."

"For me?" Dorrie eagerly took the bag and quickly pulled out the teddy bear and hugged it tightly.

I felt obligated to create an excuse for the childish present. "You needed someone to hug you yesterday when you were going through that. Next time you're in pain, Mrs. Holmes, you won't be alone."

Dorrie started to cry. I comforted her, thinking she was reliving the recent crisis. After she blew her nose and dabbed her tears, she looked at me, still clutching the teddy bear.

"Do you know that this is the first teddy bear I've ever gotten. I've always wanted one, since I was a little girl. I've given many as gifts, but never got one myself. This really means a lot to me."

Now the tears were in my eyes. I went over and gave her a hug and kiss on the cheek.

"Please call me Dorrie," she whispered in my ear as she held me tight.

She was eventually discharged, not to the dreaded nursing home, but to the home of a niece who felt she could handle her because she was able to walk around. Until the day she left, her teddy was proudly displayed on the bedside stand and she would point to her teddy bear and smile any time I walked in the room.

Dorrie's life had purpose and meaning. For months, she was a wonderful patient who allowed herself to be a teaching tool for dozens of students. For Dorrie, and the millions of others who have said "yes" when asked if a student could care for them, we owe a debt of gratitude.

* * *

Over the years it has been a joy to look up as a patient, or family member of a patient, in a health facility and realize that one of your own former students is your nurse! I have been blessed to watch them provide competent and compassionate care and for just a brief moment imagine that I played a role in that somehow. But seeing "my" students in so many different places, I realize now what unique talents they each brought with them to our school. Each had a calling to use "their gifts" in ways I had never even imagined for them.

The best bedside nurses went on to clinical positions all over the area with many, like Dale, in leadership roles. The Bill's of the world found their passion in cardiology or the emergency room. The Russell's and Danielle's combined their nursing degrees with management degrees or went on with their own nursing education. The Linda's used their nursing background in unique ways, like holistic health centers.

Caitlin never made it all the way through the program, despite her will and motivation to succeed, she remained unsafe clinically. As faculty we are called to be gatekeepers for the profession. That is never an easy message to deliver. Often students like Caitlin try to get through LPN school or just wind up as wonderful nurses' aides.

Meanwhile, Amy managed to slither through the program just above the bar, motivated by the money and the promise of employment. I hear she left the field and took a job without patient contact in an insurance company within the year. Students like Amy never last long in nursing. There can be no personal job satisfaction in a job poorly done.

Nursing at the RN level is not for everyone.

* * *

The time had come for me to move on from teaching in a classroom. My ongoing education and experiences had proven time and time again that I was ready to be the diagnostician and decision maker for the patient. I explored the idea of medical school, but after much soul searching and discussions with close friends, I chose to put the emotional needs of my three children and my spouse first and forever closed the door to that dream. I had already invested in a Master's degree in nursing so I chose to stay on that same road and added a post-master's degree as a Family Nurse Practitioner.

"..for it is God who works in you to will and to act according to his good purpose."

Philippians 2:12

PART THREE:

WHAT'S IN A TITLE?

19

Beyond the Lab Coat

"Thanks doc!" the patient said as she left the exam room. Once again, I would politely explain that I was a Family Nurse Practitioner (FNP), not a doctor.

"Well, you are my doctor and I'll call you what I want", or "You should have been!", or "You're as good as any doctor I've ever had!" Phrases my FNP nurse colleagues and I heard on a regular basis.

My vast array of experiences in bedside nursing and teaching brought me well prepared for the variety of patients in the primary care setting. Life as a Nurse Practitioner in a busy primary care office in New York is the same for Medical Doctors (MDs) and Doctors of Osteopathy (DOs) as it is for Family Nurse Practitioners. FNPs are licensed and educated to do everything MDs and DOs can do in this setting, and without supervision. Like all "providers" at this level of care, FNPs are responsible to provide the highest quality care, and to reach out to colleagues for advice with patients in areas outside our scope of practice or expertise. Like all primary care providers, FNP are required to know how to treat a little of everything.

There are no predictable days. Behind every door waits a new surprise: a 3 year old with a jelly bean up her nose; a 52 year old here for a sinus infection who bursts into tears because her spouse just left her; a 10 year that needs stitches in his hand; a 62 year old here for a physical whose heartburn last week was really a heart attack and he gets shipped off in an ambulance; a 16 year old girl here for a physical who has an eating disorder that she finally admits to having to you, 24 minutes into a 30 minute time slot; a 20 year old boy with genital anal warts from his boyfriend; a 50 year old follow up for hypertension and hyperlipidemia; an 86 year old woman you need to convince to go to a nursing home;

a 2 day old infant who isn't latching well onto mom's breast; a 42 year old obese out of control diabetic who shares how she doesn't thinks she really needs insulin because she started exercising and eating right (again) just last week. Only ten more patients and the day will be over.

In between visits, we are expected to address phone calls, review test results and specialist's consultation reports, complete patient forms, and coordinate care for several thousand patients while covering for other physicians. With every patient encounter and every paper comes a decision: acknowledge, sign, change therapy, or answer a question. It is estimated that primary care providers make over a hundred critical decisions a day. Days that never end on time. And with the mandatory adoption of computerized records, depending on your program, several hours of documentation time was likely added to the day's workload.

With only 15-30 minutes for a visit there is often only enough time for a patient patch job. But patients don't come for band-aids, they come for solutions. They often would tell me, "I came because I knew *you* would take the time to sort this out and solve this for me!" Like the 42 year old woman with red stool that went through a negative gastro-intestinal work-up that I realized was caused from her eating beets. Or the assembly line of migraine patients that were able to resolve their headaches with either new pillows, changes in light bulbs at work, or raising the height of their keyboards. There were countless patients with knee or hip pain, returning from their orthopedic surgeons with a negative MRI report in hand, that would clear up once I showed them a few simple stretching exercises or how to stand or sit differently at work. My favorite was the woman with unrelenting tendonitis in her arm that no one could figure out where it was coming from. When I realized she was a school bus driver, I asked her to show me how she opened the bus door to let the kids on. As she raised her arm and reached out, simulating the motion, she yelped, "Ow!" Now we could fix it. Because nurses are taught to focus on the whole person in the context of their social and cultural environment, FNPs are a perfect match for primary care settings.

A wonderful part of being a FNP is the "family" part, the relationships formed over the years. I had the honor and privilege to cuddle dozens of newborn babies, then watch them head off to kindergarten and become dancers, singers, and sports enthusiasts. I watched as the kids with the tiny legs swinging from the exam table grew into full size men with beards, taking their first jobs post-college. And I watched pig-tailed girls and freckled boys grow up to become nurses like me! I got to know their siblings, their parents, their ex-parents, their grandparents, their neighbors and their friends. I was there for their traumas, emotional and physical. They shared their deepest secrets with me and allowed me to help them negotiate through the stressors of growing up. I kept a few from quitting college, prevented a few suicides, reversed a few dangerous eating patterns in the nick of time, and helped to heal a lot of broken relationships.

You do develop favorites, and interestingly enough it is not always the "perfect" patients. Some of my favorites have been my most non-compliant patients. I had several that wouldn't stop smoking, despite severe lung disease. I had one who was a diabetic that came very regularly for appointments, but wouldn't stop eating donuts for breakfast because she didn't want to lose weight and look wrinkly! Another favorite was a cirrhosis patient who gave up alcohol for several years but who one day left me a voice mail to tell me that he had found a cure for his shakes; he had drunk a beer and he felt great! Perhaps it was the twinkle in their eyes as they told me the raw truth that I came to respect and appreciate.

I had several favorite albeit really stinky patients over the years that my aides would gag just putting in the rooms. These individuals and families were clearly unaware of the aroma that surrounded them due to failure to clean themselves or their clothes. They helped me keep my life in perspective, to count my own blessings. Their lives were riddled with drama, trauma, and consequences of either bad choices or circumstances outside their control. Vietnam vets still jumping at any little sound. Third generation poverty. Children whose parents had used drugs, leaving them with learning disabilities and a life-long sentence of low income. Or people who were just born without motivation and drive, and despite opportunities, had nothing but unfulfilled dreams. When I challenged myself to get to know the story and strengths of the person behind the aroma, to see them through God's eyes, he never disappointed me.

My absolute favorites were the patients that if I had met under any other circumstances could have been my best friends. Crazy creative people, fellow writers, therapists, thinkers. All of us on separate journeys, just crossing paths. As a professional, I was the one who was supposed to be there for them, but many times, they were there for me. I can never thank them enough for the moments shared.

Naturally, there were a few patients that no one liked. Fortunately for the Hippocratic Oath, these patients still got good care! Misbehaving patients were discharged, some with police escorts. My shortest patient relationship was two minutes. He started screaming at me when I asked him what medicines he was taking.

"I don't think this relationship is going to work," I suggested as I left the room. He was not charged for the visit.

Over the years, it became apparent to me that the majority of my patient's symptoms were self-induced, stress related, or the result of untreated anxiety or depression. Sometimes a patient's problem was obvious to everyone but them. Sometimes a patient's real problem was locked inside where no one could see it; an axe buried deep, grinding away at a person's inner health. No matter what treatment was used, these patients would not get better unless their underlying emotional issues were revealed and validated so that all that negative energy could be redirected in positive, healthy ways.

Megan was in my office frequently, always armed with a checklist of the latest body symptoms plaguing her for the past month such as headaches, muscle aches, diarrhea, abdominal pain, or intermittent rashes. She would persist with her presentation until some bloodwork was drawn, convinced that this time her illness would reveal itself for others to see. Megan was not responding to any combination of drugs, diets, or exercise program.

Megan would share her symptoms intermixed with her stressors, a sign to me that the source for her physical symptoms was her emotional distress. "My headaches have been out of control since my son enlisted in the military - still I've been eating the diet like you taught me, but the other day when my ex stopped by, and well that didn't go well with my daughter, that